T0320960

Addiction Potential
of Abused Drugs
and Drug Classes

The *Advances in Alcohol & Substance Abuse* series:

- *Recent Advances in the Biology of Alcoholism*
- *The Effects of Maternal Alcohol and Drug Abuse on the Newborn*
- *Evaluation of Drug Treatment Programs*
- *Current Controversies in Alcoholism*
- *Federal Priorities in Funding Alcohol and Drug Abuse Programs*
- *Psychosocial Constructs of Alcoholism and Substance Abuse*
- *The Addictive Behaviors*
- *Conceptual Issues in Alcoholism and Substance Abuse*
- *Dual Addiction: Pharmacological Issues in the Treatment of Concomitant Alcoholism and Drug Abuse*
- *Cultural and Sociological Aspects of Alcoholism and Substance Abuse*
- *Alcohol and Drug Abuse in the Affluent*
- *Alcohol and Substance Abuse in Adolescence*
- *Controversies in Alcoholism and Substance Abuse*
- *Alcohol and Substance Abuse in Women and Children*
- *Cocaine: Pharmacology, Addiction, and Therapy*
- *Children of Alcoholics*
- *Pharmacological Issues in Alcohol and Substance Abuse*
- *AIDS and Substance Abuse*
- *Alcohol Research from Bench to Bedside*
- *Addiction Potential of Abused Drugs and Drug Classes*

Addiction Potential of Abused Drugs and Drug Classes

Carlton K. Erickson, PhD
Martin A. Javors, PhD
William W. Morgan, PhD
Guest Editors

Barry Stimmel, MD
Editor

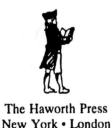

The Haworth Press
New York • London

Addiction Potential of Abused Drugs and Drug Classes has also been published as *Advances in Alcohol & Substance Abuse*, Volume 9, Numbers 1/2 1990.

The Haworth Press, Inc., 10 Alice Street, Binghamton, NY 13904-1580
EUROSPAN/Haworth, 3 Henrietta Street, London WC2E 8LU England

Library of Congress Cataloging-in-Publication Data

Addiction potential of abused drugs and drug classes / guest editors, Carlton K. Erickson, Martin A. Javors, William W. Morgan; editor, Barry Stimmel.
    p. cm.
    "Has also been published as Advances in alcohol and substance abuse, volume 9, numbers 1/2, 1990"—T.p. verso.
    Includes bibliographical references.
    ISBN 0-86656-975-8
    1. Drug abuse. 2. Psychotropic drugs—Physiological effect. I. Erickson, Carlton K. II. Javors, Martin A. III. Morgan, William W., 1945- . IV. Stimmel, Barry.
    [DNLM: 1. Street Drugs—pharmacology. 2. Substance Dependence. W1 AD432 v. 9 no. 1/2 / WM 270 A2239]
RC564.A285   1990
616.86'071—dc20
DNLM/DLC
for Library of Congress   90-4639
                                      CIP

Addiction Potential of Abused Drugs and Drug Classes

Advances in Alcohol & Substance Abuse
Volume 9, Numbers 1/2

CONTENTS

∞   ALL HAWORTH BOOKS & JOURNALS
     ARE PRINTED ON CERTIFIED
     ACID-FREE PAPER

ABOUT THE GUEST EDITORS

Carlton K. Erickson, PhD, is the Parke-Davis Centennial Professor of Pharmacology in the College of Pharmacy, University of Texas at Austin, Texas. He is currently Head of the Alcohol and Drug Abuse Research Program at the University of Texas. Dr. Erickson is nationally recognized for his research on the effects of alcohol on neurotransmitters, and he has intense interests in scientific communication and public education concerning drug abuse and alcoholism. Dr. Erickson received a BS in Pharmacy from Ferris State College in Big Rapids, Michigan in 1961, and a PhD in Pharmacology and Toxicology from Purdue University in 1965.

Martin A. Javors, PhD, is Associate Professor in the Departments of Psychiatry and Pharmacology at the University of Texas Health Science Center at San Antonio, Texas. During the past several years, Dr. Javors has studied the metabolic control of intracellular calcium ion concentration by membrane receptors and the role of the calcium ion as an intracellular second messenger in secretory cells, especially the blood platelet. He has studied these biochemical and physiological aspects of calcium ion metabolism and their relationship to alcoholism, depression, and schizophrenia. Dr. Javors received a BS in Pharmacy from the University of Texas at Austin in 1967, and a PhD in Pharmacy (Biochemical Pharmacology) from the University of Colorado at Boulder in 1979.

William W. Morgan, PhD, is Professor of Neurochemistry in the Department of Cellular and Structural Biology at the University of Texas Health Science Center at San Antonio, Texas. Dr. Morgan's current research interests relate to the role of neurotransmitters in the brain in the development of barbiturate dependence and the subsequent manifestation of the barbiturate abstinence syndrome, the role of GABA and catecholamines in the regulation of vasopressin secretion from the posterior pituitary, and the molecular mechanisms involved in the tissue-specific expression of the tyrosine hydroxylase gene. Dr. Morgan received his BS degree from Indiana State University in 1966, and his PhD from Indiana University, Bloomington, Indiana in 1970.

EDITORIAL

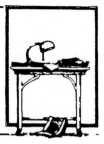

Drug Dependence: Defining the Issues

There has always been, and will continue to be, controversy over drug addiction—what it is, which drug users acquire it, what drug is most addicting, etc. Just the term "addiction" has multiple meanings to the general public, to the user, and to scientists of different backgrounds.

Carlton K. Erickson is affiliated with the Alcohol and Drug Abuse Research Program, College of Pharmacy, The University of Texas, Austin, TX 78712. Martin A. Javors is affiliated with the Department of Psychiatry, The University of Texas Health Science Center, San Antonio, TX 78284. William W. Morgan is affiliated with the Department of Cellular and Structural Biology, The University of Texas Health Science Center, San Antonio, TX 78284.

This volume was partially funded through a contract from the Texas Commission on Alcohol and Drug Abuse, Austin, TX.

1

The papers in this volume clarify, in contemporary terminology, the state of addiction liability of the drugs which are most abused today. Nine drugs and drug classes have been chosen for review. Authors have meshed their research expertise with the available scientific literature to evaluate those factors which contribute to the addictive qualities of drugs. For operational definitions they have used a recent article published in the Journal of the American Medical Association which was written to clarify drug abuse and addiction terminology based upon a Delphi survey of substance abuse experts.[1] We further refined five definitions felt to be critically important for this book:

Abuse — This term is used when drug taking is harmful but not so extreme as to achieve the criteria for dependence.

(Drug) dependence — A physiological state of adaptation to a drug, often characterized by the development of tolerance to drug effects, and the emergence of a withdrawal syndrome during prolonged abstinence.

Psychological dependence — This describes chronic drug-taking behavior presumably related to the reinforcing (rewarding) effects of the drug. The term involves "chronic and compulsive" drug-taking and "impaired control over drug-taking."

(Drug) addiction — This is a global description of a pattern of chronic, compulsive drug-taking behavior which is harmful.

One other point regarding definitions needs to be made. While "addiction" is always "abuse," the reverse is not always true. Most of the authors of the following papers describe "drug addicts and abusers," suggesting that they are two separate groups of drug-takers. In some cases (as with alcohol and perhaps nicotine), there is such a spectrum of drug use in duration and amount, and in the presence or absence of dependence, that a case can be made that a subgroup of drug-takers can abuse a drug without showing all the signs of addiction. It would follow, then, that "compulsive loss of control" over drug-taking would characterize the true addictive state, which is also analogous to the "disease" of addiction. The controversial nature of "addiction as disease" has been recently discussed,[2] and regardless of whether one believes this definition of drug addiction as a disease, it should be clear that drug abusers need to be treated clinically in a different manner than drug addicts. The usefulness of acknowledging such a difference is seen when the public, including those who vote for or against drug abuse research funds, understands that addiction is a mystery which research can solve. Furthermore, the solution can come about without an attack on the one-martini or one-glass-of-wine lunch, which some may classify as "abuse," but not addiction.

The "loss of control," and "spectrum of euphoria to craving" concept is best described (for cocaine) in the paper by Dackis and Gold. This description covers the neuroanatomical and neurochemical bases of psychological dependence, which is the greatest contributing factor to drug addiction. If "craving" or "loss of control" is great for a particular drug, the addiction liability is also great. On the other hand, a drug's "abuse potential" is primarily based upon pleasurable feelings produced by the drug, society's attitude toward users of the drug, and the toxicity (or lack thereof) of the drug.

We believe that a particular drug's "addiction potential" is more important than its "abuse potential" in the drug's impact on society and medicine. We have taken this into consideration in our summary listing of drugs which are addicting, given here in order of decreasing addiction potential:

1. central stimulants (esp. cocaine)
2. opiates
3. alcohol
4. sedative-hypnotics
5. nicotine
6. anxiolytics
7. marihuana
8. inhalants and anesthetics
9. PCP and hallucinogens

Another, more sensible, listing would have been to rank order the drugs and drug classes based upon the percentage of users who become dependent upon the drug ("dependence liability"). However, these data are not available for all drug classes. For alcohol, the often-cited percentage is 10% (i.e., 1 in 10 alcohol drinkers become "dependent"), while Dackis and Gold indicate that 85% of users who called the national cocaine help line "felt out of control." If such figures were available for other addicting drugs, a rank ordering of dependence liability would be more accurate than the list given above. Furthermore, such percentages would be very helpful to the general public to understand the likelihood of becoming dependent on drugs. It is important to keep in mind, however, that within each drug class (e.g., opiates), some drugs (e.g., heroin) are known to produce dependence more readily than other drugs (e.g., methadone).

The elements identified by several authors in their papers as being related to addiction potential are: (1) *craving*, a strong desire to take the drug for its euphorigenic effects or, possibly, to avoid the effects of not taking it; (2) *length of use*, the amount of time the person has been taking the drug for non-therapeutic purposes; (3) *denial*, the continued use of a drug despite its harmful effects, including health and legal reasons (denial includes concealing drug use from others); (4) *recidivism*, the return to abuse of a drug after a period of successful abstinence; (5) *dependence*, a state in which the abuser requires the drug for normal life function, but not to the stage where the drug has become the paramount factor in life; (6) *rate of progression*, the amount of time from first use to dependence on a drug (for example, the rate is rapid with cocaine but slow with alcohol); (7) *the obsession element*, involving the stage of addiction where use and obtaining the drug become the paramount preoccupation of the abuser, even to the point of harm to one's relationship with family, job, friends, etc.; and (8) *sociological elements*, involving factors such as social acceptance and peer pressure that motivate a person to use the drug. Some of these factors may be absent with certain drugs but are certainly present when considering the entire spectrum of addiction.

Several authors discuss the positive and negative reinforcement qualities which make drugs rewarding. These concepts are so important that they are worth mentioning here. Positive reinforcement is a situation where a drug produces euphoria or a sense of well-being in a person looking for a drug "high." Cocaine is an excellent example of a drug which produces positive reinforcement. Negative reinforcement is seen when a drug is used to prevent or overcome dysphoria: anxiety, pain, depression, boredom, etc. Thus, anxiolytics relieve anxiety and produce negative reinforcement. In actuality, most abused drugs produce positive or negative reinforcement depending upon the expectations of the user, the environment, dose, and many other factors. Both positive and negative reinforcement are associated with the early, causative effects of drug use and abuse. When dependence occurs, drugs are taken primarily to prevent craving or withdrawal (negative reinforcement).

As might be expected, there are several topics which are not covered in this volume. Although the acquired immune deficiency syndrome (AIDS) is an important topic related to drug abuse, there is no indication that AIDS affects the addiction potential of any drug class. Theoretically, AIDS could affect the immune system of drug users so that the susceptibility to drug dependence might change. However, there is no solid scientific evidence to support such an hypothesis. On another front, some centrally active drugs such as caffeine, antidepressants, and antipsychotic agents are not discussed. Until recently, there was no concern over dependency on these drugs, and available evidence now suggests that these drugs do not produce clinically dangerous loss of control or compulsive drug-seeking behavior. However, they can be abused (as can laxatives and cold medicines, for example), and there may even be significant withdrawal in some cases (for caffeine, excellent reviews[3,4] are available). Nevertheless, we have chosen not to cover the lesser-abused centrally-active drugs in this issue. Finally, the neurochemical and metabolic mechanisms of physical dependence and tolerance are not covered. There is a wealth of scientific literature on these topics (especially with ethanol and opiates), and that literature does not need to be reviewed to understand the addictive potential of abused drugs.

The paper on alcohol by Lewis briefly mentions the two major subtypes of alcoholics. It is likely that drug addictions in general will ultimately be subtyped in the clinical literature, based upon several factors: cause of dependence, psychological or social characteristics, or severity of addiction. Such possibilities are exciting, for typology of disease allows more specific and individualized treatments to be designed and implemented.

It is anticipated that the papers in this volume will increase the awareness of scientists, clinicians, administrators, and others of the relative addiction liabilities of various drugs and drug classes that are abused. It is also important, however, to highlight those areas where more work is needed in order to understand how individual drugs affect the processes of dependence, tolerance, and addiction, so that adequate treatment of these disorders can be discovered. It is clear, for example, that cocaine addiction is among the most difficult disorders to treat, simply because we do not yet understand the complete psychological, social, and neurochemical causes of cocaine addiction and relapse. With future research, better and more cost-effective treatment and prevention strategies should become available.

Future research on alcohol and other drug abuse is threatened by the meager federal support available for such research. In FY 1987, for example, the National Institute on Drug Abuse (NIDA) received less than $124 million for research into the causes and consequences of all drug abuse other than alcohol. The National Institute on Alcohol Abuse and Alcoholism (NIAAA) the same year received less than $72 million for research on alcohol abuse and alcoholism, arguably the nation's second-leading disease based upon incidence and cost to the public. Compared to the over $1.3 billion for cancer research and $800 million for heart and cardiovascular disease research in FY 1987, it appears that the rate of acquisition of new knowledge about alcohol and other drug abuse and addiction will be relatively slow in the foreseeable future. A large influx of federal dollars into alcohol and other drug abuse research is certainly required to fill the knowledge gaps that are apparent throughout the papers that follow.

Carlton K. Erickson, PhD
Martin A. Javors, PhD
William W. Morgan, PhD

REFERENCES

1. Rinaldi RC, Steindler EM, Wilford BB, Goodwin D. Clarification and standardization of substance abuse terminology. J Am Med Assoc 1988; 259: 555-7.

2. Scott N. The Fingarette fallacies. Alc Addict 1988; July-August: 17-19.

3. Griffiths RR, Woodson PP. Caffeine physical dependence: A review of human and laboratory animal studies. Psychopharmacology 1988; 94:437-51.

4. Griffiths RR, Woodson PP. Reinforcing effects of caffeine in humans. J Pharmacol Exp Ther 1988; 246:21-9.

Addictiveness of Central Stimulants

Charles A. Dackis, MD
Mark S. Gold, MD

SUMMARY. Central stimulants have been abused since their inception and we are currently in the midst of a cocaine epidemic that challenges our resources and capabilities. Through their actions on powerful endogenous reward centers, central stimulants produce intense euphoria that reinforces subsequent usage and eventual dependence. Considerable evidence indicates that the activation of dopamine circuits mediates stimulant reward. With regard to cocaine, it has been hypothesized that depletion of central dopamine leads to craving. Euphoria and craving, the key dynamics of stimulant addiction, may therefore result largely from neurochemical alterations of dopamine systems in the brain's reward center. Progressive deterioration of the stimulant addict involving medical, psychiatric, and psychosocial impairment occurs rapidly, underscoring the addiction potential of these agents. Tolerance, sensitization and withdrawal phenomena are discussed from clinical and neurochemical perspectives.

INTRODUCTION

Central stimulants have fascinated and entrapped people ever since their euphorogenic properties were first experienced. There have been numerous epidemics with cocaine and amphetamine, occurring during different time periods and within various cultures. Nonetheless, persistent minimization of their addictiveness and medical hazards endures. The addictive potential of central stimu-

Charles A. Dackis and Mark S. Gold are affiliated with the Research Facilities at Hampton Hospital, Rancocas, NJ, and Fair Oaks Hospital, Summit, NJ, respectively.

9

lants is minimized for several reasons. These agents do not produce the dramatic withdrawal syndromes seen with opiates, alcohol, and sedative/hypnotics. Since there is an exaggerated importance placed on "physical withdrawal" in our present conceptualization of addiction, the "mild" withdrawal syndromes seen with stimulants has led to a view that they are merely "psychologically addictive." Furthermore, stimulant use is typically characterized by binges, with intermittent drug-free days. Since stimulant addicts may not use every day, they may be seen as less addicted. Until recently these conceptions have been widely accepted by the medical community. With cocaine, the tremendous cost limits access for many individuals, precluding the nightmarish addiction in many that evolves with unlimited supply. Finally, the marketing of cocaine is greatly facilitated by its safe mythology, so that both dealers and addicts are quick to promote the idea that this stimulant is safe and non-addictive.

The central stimulants that are significantly abused at present are amphetamine (dextroamphetamine and methamphetamine) and cocaine. Methylphenidate is widely used in the treatment of adolescents, and its abuse potential will be briefly reviewed. This paper will largely focus on cocaine since we are currently immersed in a cocaine epidemic, and its abuse involves the greatest clinical problem of the group. Differences encountered in defining addiction to amphetamine and other stimulants will be highlighted when applicable.

Several crucial questions about stimulants will be addressed in this article. Does stimulant dependence share sufficient characteristics with addiction to other substances to warrant its inclusion in the broad category of addictive illness? Is stimulant dependence progressive and, if so, how does the rate of progression compare with that seen with other agents? Should treatment approaches differ with stimulant abusers? Are there important reversible or irreversible neurochemical changes that occur with chronic exposure to stimulants? These questions will be examined by reviewing the epidemiology, clinical nature, neurochemistry and repercussions of stimulant dependence.

EPIDEMIOLOGICAL CONSIDERATIONS

A number of epidemiological facts support the addictiveness of cocaine and amphetamine. From a historical perspective, there have been several cocaine epidemics in Europe and the United States around the turn of the century. Each ended when cocaine's addictiveness became so obvious that the pool of first time users dissipated, and the prevalence of addicts subsequently waned. Amphetamines created epidemics in Japan, Sweden and Denmark in the 1950's and in the United States during the 1960's when their hazards, exemplified by the street slogan, "speed kills," were similarly appreciated. The controversy over stimulant addictiveness has therefore varied with the mystique surrounding particular agents and the time period in question.

Surveys of cocaine addicts are an informative if not entirely rigorous means of assessing addictiveness. A recent study found that 74% of random callers to a national cocaine help line (800-Cocaine) felt addicted, 85% felt out of control and could not refuse cocaine if offered, and 76% were unable to stop use for one month.[1] In addition, 75% described withdrawal symptoms and 73% preferred cocaine over food, family and all other recreational activities. Adverse psychosocial effects of cocaine were also evident. Callers reported dealing to support their habit (47%), stealing from family members (42%), assuming debt due to cocaine (57%), and losing their spouse as a result of the addiction (33%). Loss of job (15%) and arrest for possession or sale (14%) was also reported.[1] Nine out of ten callers reported adverse emotional or physical consequences of their cocaine use. In addition, the progression of psychosocial deterioration with cocaine was more rapid than that seen with other substances of abuse.[1]

THE CLINICAL NATURE OF STIMULANT ADDICTION

The major forces that drive all forms of drug addiction are craving and drug-induced euphoria. As will be discussed later, central stimulants are extremely selective and powerful activators of endogenous reward centers. Based on animal self-administration studies, stimulants are the most rewarding of all drugs. The process of stimulant addiction begins with the pleasurable experience of stimulant reward. The reason for initial use, such as curiosity, peer pressure, boredom or adventurism, is of secondary importance to the rewarding experience. The memory of stimulant euphoria then serves as a positive reinforcer, making repeated use very likely. Clinicians who treat stimulant addicts should never underestimate the power of stimulant euphoria as a motivator of behavior. As stimulant use is repeated, craving evolves as the other major force involved in the dynamics of addiction. Craving for stimulants acts as a negative reinforcer for stimulant use, just as thirst reinforces fluid intake. In fact, it is very likely that the same reward centers that mediate the drives of thirst, hunger and libido are involved in stimulant euphoria and craving. As the cycle of craving and euphoria becomes increasingly entrenched and uncontrollable, the thin line is crossed into addiction. At this point, the addict begins to tolerate greater hazards associated with stimulant use, using denial to justify progressive deterioration of health and psychosocial functioning. The amount and frequency of use increases, financial penalties of addiction are accepted and overlooked, and the procurement and use of stimulants becomes the addict's first priority.

Stimulant addiction might seem illogical until the primary organ of involvement is better understood. Just as pneumonia affects the lungs, stimulants affect and disrupt endogenous reward centers in the brain. These structures have evolved to insure that survival needs like feeding, procreation and fluid intake are fulfilled. Considerable evidence supports the notion that the pharmacological and neurochemical actions of stimulants on endogenous "pleasure centers" generate drug euphoria[2] and craving,[3] particularly through the stimulation and depletion of central dopamine (DA) pathways. Since these natural drive systems are acted upon by central stimulants, stimulant craving may be conceptualized as an "acquired drive" driven by powerful, genetically encoded reward centers in the midbrain. The involvement of endogenous reward centers explains why animals self-administer stimulants to the point of death,[4] and addicts gradually lose control over the cycle of euphoria and craving. Interestingly, natural driven reduction (feeding, mating, drinking) satiates the active drive, but stimulant use seems to induce or potentiate the drive to consume more stimulants. This phenomenon of impaired satiation comprises an essential clinical and neurochemical dynamic of the addiction process and may be due to DA depletion by stimulants.[1]

Euphoria

Since stimulant euphoria is a major reinforcer of this addiction, it deserves some descriptive attention. In blind studies, stimulant addicts are not able to distinguish the subjective effects of cocaine from amphetamine, and animals readily substitute methylphenidate, methylamphetamine, d-amphetamine and L-amphetamine for cocaine in self-administration studies.[5] It is therefore reasonable to generalize the subjective experience of cocaine to these other central stimulants.

Intravenous or intrapulmonary administration of cocaine produces an intense "rush" of pleasure lasting several seconds and followed by persistent but lower level euphoria. The intensity of the cocaine "high" is illustrated by the fact that spontaneous ejaculation without genital stimulation has been reported after intravenous cocaine administration.[6] Stimulant intoxication includes euphoria, increased energy and alertness, enhanced sensory experience and libido, and elevated self-confidence. Physiological effects of hypertension, tachycardia, diaphoresis, mydriasis and hyperkinesis coincide with the subjective state, and with blood levels of the drug. The initial pleasure of cocaine intoxication is fleeting, and euphoria gives way to irritability, "crashing" mood, and craving for more cocaine as the positive subjective effects wear off. In addition to craving, the memory of euphoria reinforces subsequent drug use. Stimulant euphoria, which is far outside the range of normal subjective states, appears to have a strong physiological basis since its description is fairly constant among addicts. Also supporting a biological basis of this state is the fact that amphetamine euphoria is blocked in human subjects pretreated with DA antagonists.[7]

Stimulant addicts seeking treatment often state they no longer derive as much or any pleasure from their drug of choice. This phenomenon sometimes reflects their denial, but also relates to the fact that stimulant intoxication may become less pleasurable as the addiction progresses. This problem often leads addicts to increase their frequency of use or change the route of administration (injecting or smoking) in an attempt to recapture the old "highs" of their earlier experience.[8] The loss of pleasure underscores two crucial points. First, some degree of disruption in the pleasure centers probably occurs to explain the diminished potency of stimulants over time. Secondly, since stimulant addicts frequently complain of generalized boredom and disinterest, cocaine exposure may impair their overall capacity for enjoyment.

Craving

Craving comprises the other major reinforcer in the dynamics of stimulant addiction. A crucial aspect of any addiction, craving develops gradually over time and leads directly to continued use or recidivism through negative reinforcement. As previously mentioned, craving for stimulants may be viewed as an "acquired" drive that is similar and perhaps more intense than hunger, thirst and sex drive. In fact, the DA systems affected by stimulants are also involved in the mediation of these survival drives,[2] explaining how the brain may be "tricked" into thinking a survival need is being met through the use of stimulants. The degree by which addicts choose their drug over survival drives is actually a useful clinical indicator of addiction severity. The strongest survival drive is undoubtedly for oxygen, and few suffocating addicts would choose their drug over air. However, addicts and laboratory animals routinely choose stimulants over sex, food and water.[9]

Stimulant craving can be separated into at least three subtypes. *Acute craving* begins minutes after the intoxication state begins to wear off. At this point the user is experiencing a rapid drop euphoria that gives way to irritability, depression, and a desperate urge to avert the evolving dysphoria through the use of more drug. This acute craving serves to perpetuate the stimulant binge and explains why addicts usually consume their entire available supply. *Intermediate craving* typically begins after the cocaine (or amphetamine) "crash" has resolved, and decreases irregularly over a period of several weeks. Unfortunately, most cocaine addicts are unable or unwilling to remain abstinent for several weeks. Abstinent addicts are also vulnerable to *provoked craving*, which is triggered by conditioned cues of the drug environment. Freebase pipes, mirrors, or the actual sight of cocaine are capable of producing intense craving,[10] even after long periods of abstinence. This third type of craving is addressed by the treatment strategy of avoiding "people, places and things" capable of its induction.

Tolerance and Sensitization

Tolerance is defined as a physiological adaptation to the effects of a drug that is manifested by a requirement for increased dosage to maintain the same intensity and duration of the drug's effect. With central stimulants, tolerance is somewhat complicated. Certain actions, such as epileptogenesis, involve reverse tolerance, or sensitization. For instance, daily administration of a fixed dose of cocaine will eventually produce seizures consistently, but only after several days. This phenomenon, known as "kindling," occurs as the brain becomes sensitized to cocaine.[11] Sensitization may also occur with psychotic symptoms such as hallucinations and paranoia, and with cardiac arrhythmias. Sensitization to pharmacological effects does not occur with opiates or sedative/hypnotic drugs, where tolerance is the rule. The mechanism of sensitization appears to involve the supersensitivity of adrenergic receptors in response to presynaptic depletion.[1]

Tolerance also occurs with stimulants. Tolerance to stimulant euphoria is readily described by addicts, leading them to increase consumption and often switch to intrapulmonary or intravenous routes of administration.[8] Tolerance also develops with respect to the effects of hyperthermia, anorexia, hypertension and nonadrenaline release. Tolerance to the euphorogenic effects of stimulants overrides sensitization to adverse effects because, with drug addicts, positive reinforcement is more powerful than the deterrent of medical hazards. In fact, addiction is often defined as the compulsive use of a drug without regard to adverse consequences.

Impaired Satiation

It is useful at this time to focus on an important aspect of cocaine use, namely the satiation of cocaine craving. Since we have already compared cocaine craving with survival drives, an examination of important differences might be helpful. A normal drive (hunger, thirst, sex drive) is satiated by the corresponding consumatory event. However, satiation does not follow a linear pattern since initial consumption stimulates a greater albeit temporary craving. The first few morsels of food are pleasurable, but initially stimulate even greater hunger and more consumption. A popular potato chip advertisement dares us to "eat only one." Eventually, with enough food intake, hunger is alleviated (although bulimics show impairment in this satiation mechanism).

With cocaine, satiation either fails to occur or develops only after the addict has collapsed into exhaustion. This pattern is similarly seen in animal studies where self-administration of central stimulants continues to the point of collapse, seizures or death.[4] The phenomenon of impaired satiation is poorly understood but probably exists in all forms of substance abuse. Alcoholics have much greater resistance to alcohol craving before their first drink, after which subsequent intake proceeds in an uncontrollable fashion. The satiation mechanism is especially impaired with stimulants, leading to the characteristic pattern of bingeing.

Satiation is the opposite of craving. Neuronal mechanisms of satiation have evolved to limit needless behavior and dangerous intake of food and fluids. Subsequent sections will explore the role of DA circuits in the mediation of cocaine craving. It has been hypothesized that craving (lack of satiation) results from DA depletion.[3] If DA circuits are normally involved in the mechanism of satiation, their depletion by stimulants might explain how satiation goes awry, and addiction progresses over time.

Stimulant Withdrawal

Aside from alternating periods of euphoria and craving, stimulants are capable of producing withdrawal, or "crashing" states. Stimulant withdrawal was largely overlooked for years, reinforcing the false notion that only "psychological" dependence occurs with these agents. The stimulant withdrawal syndrome, first described with amphetamines,[12] persists one to three days and includes fatigue, depression, amotivation, hypersomnia, decreased libido, and hyperphagia. Interestingly, the cocaine withdrawal syndrome (cocaine "crash") does not usually include the craving for cocaine, which instead tends to return several days later.[13] "Crashing" symptoms are not as dramatic as withdrawal syndromes associated with opiates or sedatives because the neurochemical basis appears to involve catecholamine depletion rather than catecholamine rebound hyperactivity.[3] Stimulant withdrawal varies with the dose, duration and frequency of abuse, much in the way opiate withdrawal varies with severity of opiate use, but probably contributes only minimally to the perpetuation of addiction since craving is seldom experienced until "crashing" symptoms have abated.

In general, the importance of physical withdrawal in the perpetuation of drug addiction is greatly overemphasized. Clinicians experienced in treating alcoholics or heroin addicts universally agree that these patients cannot be merely detoxified and expected to remain abstinent. Craving and the memory of drug euphoria will lead quickly to recidivism unless aggressive rehabilitation is also part of their clinical management. The tendency to define addiction as "psychological" or "physical" based on withdrawal syndromes is a misconception, resulting from the notion that craving and euphoria are merely "psychological" phenomena of secondary importance. Actually, the pharmacological production of euphoria and the neurochemical basis of craving *are* "physical" events in the brain, and comprise the most essential dynamics of addiction.

Progression

The next crucial clinical characteristic of stimulant addiction, and indeed all forms of drug addiction, is that of progression. The concept of progression has two features. First, there is progressive loss of control over the quantity and frequency of drug administration with resulting deterioration in medical, psychosocial, financial and occupational functioning. Secondly, there is the tendency to rapidly resume the previously attained severity of addiction even after lengthy periods of abstinence. This tendency, described in the recovery community as "getting back on the train where you got off," suggests a permanent physical derangement in addiction. Although progressive disorders are familiar in medicine, it is remarkable how poorly understood this essential feature of stimulant addiction remains.

The progressive worsening of stimulant addiction over time forms a descending spiral of craving and euphoria that results in a general deterioration of the patient's life. Denial, the tendency to ignore evolving hazards of addiction, operates to mask the engulfing power that is increasingly exerted over the addict. Drug craving and euphoria result from the activation and disruption of genetically encoded systems of reward in the brain. These systems evolved to insure survival, and are therefore (by definition) extremely powerful and compelling. Euphoria and craving overwhelm the addict's fears of catastrophe, explaining why compulsive drug use continues in spite of medical, financial, psychiatric and psychosocial hazards.

In the evaluation of addiction, the rate of progression is an important consideration. Certain substances are clearly capable of producing addiction more rapidly than others. First time users of heroin or cocaine are in more imminent danger of future addiction than they would be using marijuana, or even alcohol. Many more individuals use alcohol without the development of abuse or addiction compared to those using cocaine or heroin recreationally. In fact, clinical evidence suggests that cocaine dependence (especially "crack" or intrapulmonary administration) is more rapidly progressive than any other substance of abuse. For instance, "crack" addicts may experience the same degree of addiction and impairment in a period of months that is seen with years or decades of alcoholism. This rapidity of progression suggests that stimulants, particularly cocaine, are among the most addictive substances currently available.

HAZARDS OF CENTRAL STIMULANTS

An essential characteristic of drug addiction is the willingness to tolerate adverse effects or complications of compulsive use. Cirrhotic alcoholics and needle sharing heroin addicts frequently continue their drug use in spite of potentially fatal consequences. Similarly, stimulant dependence is associated with a number of medical, psychiatric, and psychosocial hazards that are increasingly tolerated as the cycle of addiction becomes more entrenched and uncontrollable. Through the process of denial, insidious dangers are overlooked or minimized. Denial is the hallmark of all drug addiction, manifests in a myriad of forms, and must be continually addressed during the course of treatment.

A brief description of medical complications of stimulant dependence underscores their addictive properties.[14] When the route of administration of cocaine or amphetamine is intravenous, individuals are predisposed to AIDS, hepatitis, endocarditis, pneumonia, sepsis and meningitis. Intrapulmonary administration (free-basing, or "crack" use) causes pulmonary dysfunction[15] and intranasal use leads to sinusitis, rhinitis, and perforated nasal septum.

Medically dangerous pharmacological actions of central stimulants are mostly the result of intense vasospasm, autonomic arousal, and direct toxic effects on the brain and heart. Sudden death may result from cardiac arrest, respiratory failure, malignant hyperthermia or stroke.[14] Acute myocardial infarction occurs even in the presence of normal coronary arteries, resulting from vasospasm in the presence of hypertension and increased myocardial oxygen demand.[16] Seizures have been reported in first time stimulant users. With repeated exposure to cocaine,[11] sensitization to seizures can result in status epilepticus. Intense vasospasm has been reported to cause cerebral, myocardial, intestinal and even placental infarction. Hypertension due to autonomic arousal has produced aortic rupture and cerebral hemorrhage. Emergency room visits by patients using cocaine are currently surging, dispelling the myth that it is medically safe.

Psychiatric complications of central stimulants are numerous. Acute intoxication with cocaine or amphetamine typically produces paranoia.[17] Other psychotic symptoms such as auditory, visual and somatic (formication) hallucinations and grandiose delusions may be present during intoxication.[17,18] Anxiety attacks, impulsivity, poor judgment and violence are frequently seen during acute intoxication. Stimulant withdrawal may produce incapacitating depressive symptoms associated with suicidality that last for days or weeks. Severe depression may be pre-existing, but can also result from neurochemical alterations in the mood centers or the addictive lifestyle.

In addition to medical and psychiatric hazards, stimulant addicts risk other dangers. Immersed in the drug environment, they often deal drugs and place themselves in dangerous situations. Imprisonment or murder are penalties of drug dealing. Job performance declines as addicts are typically intoxicated or experiencing withdrawal symptoms at work. Responsibility to family and friends suffers as drug procurement becomes the first priority.

The power of stimulant addiction, driven by the stimulation and depletion of endogenous "pleasure centers" in the brain, overrides the addict's survival considerations. Seemingly illogical pursuit of dangerous drug experiences becomes understandable in the context of deranged survival systems in the brain. The cycle of craving and euphoria, once established and entrenched, progresses in an uncontrollable fashion with stimulant addicts, in a similar but often more rapid progression compared with other addictive drugs of abuse. This explains the historical epidemics that have been recorded with central stimulants, as well as the seemingly insatiable appetite for these substances. The next section will review preclinical studies of stimulant action on the brain's reward centers, and the surprisingly rigorous administration of these drugs by animals.

PRECLINICAL STUDIES
SUPPORTING STIMULANT DEPENDENCY

A vast body of animal literature demonstrates that central stimulants can produce profound drug dependency, and that these agents are more addictive than all other classes of drugs.[1,2] Although animal researchers initially defined central stimulants as agents that produce forward locomotion in animals, a unifying definition of their rewarding action was proposed by Wise and Bozarth as the ability to activate DA circuits in the brain.[2] This important discovery is based largely on studies of stimulant self-administration by animals, which has become the preclinical standard for determining a new drug's abuse potential. Self-administration of a drug indicates rewarding activity, presumably through the stimulation of endogenous "pleasure" centers in the brain. Since animal reward is the logical equivalent of drug-induced euphoria in humans, and euphoria is a major clinical reinforcer and determinant of addiction, the assessment of self-administration data is a crucial means of measuring addictiveness in the present discussion.

Animals self-administer cocaine and amphetamine to the point of serious toxicity or death, and in preference to food, water and mating.[9] Stimulants are vigorously self-administered by all species tested, and with greater tenacity and frequency than other classes of drugs, including opiates, sedatives, and alcohol.[2,9] In fact, animals are much more likely to self-administer cocaine than heroin to the point of death. Animal studies therefore reveal that central stimulants have profound and obvious abuse potential.

Preclinical data convincingly implicate DA neurons in the mediation of stimulant reward.[2] The central stimulants discussed in this chapter (cocaine, amphetamines, methylphenidate) block the reuptake of DA from the synapse, producing an acute increase in DA neurotransmission. The activation of DA circuits has been hypothesized as a primary component of the circuitry involved in stimulant reward.[2] Self-administration of central stimulants by animals[19] and amphetamine euphoria in humans[7] are blocked or attenuated by pretreatment with selective DA receptor antagonists, while pretreatment by specific norepinephrine (NE) agents do not attenuate self-administration of stimulants. Interestingly, specific DA agonists such as apomorphine, bromocriptine and piribedil have some amphetamine-like rewarding action,[2] but not nearly to the extent seen with amphetamine, methylphenidate and cocaine.[5] The blockade of DA reuptake is more rewarding than direct postsynaptic DA receptor stimulation. This finding necessitates a refinement of the original theory that reward depends on the activation of DA circuits,[2] and implies an important presynaptic DA mechanism. Pharmacological studies do however support the notion that stimulant reward is mediated by DA systems in the brain.

Anatomical evidence also implicates DA structures in the mediation of stimulant reward. The ventral tegmentum, which is richly endowed with DA cell groups, supports both electrical and direct stimulant self-administration.[2] This region is also precisely where reward fibers of the medial forebrain bundle terminate. Lesioning of ventral tegmentum projections eliminates its ability to support electrical and stimulant self-administration. Similarly, neurotoxic lesioning of the nucleus accumbens attenuates the direct self-administration of cocaine and amphetamine into this limbic DA structure.[20] Extensive anatomical evidence supporting the role of DA structures in stimulant reward has been reviewed elsewhere.[1,21]

Since DA circuits mediate stimulant reward, acute and chronic actions of stimulants on these circuits should be examined to understand the neurochemistry of stimulant addiction. Several lines of evidence now indicate that chronic stimulant exposure leads to DA depletion. Animals subjected to chronic cocaine administration show increased DA receptor binding[22] and increased tyrosine hydroxylase activity,[1] which are compensatory responses to functional DA depletion. Even the direct measurement of brain DA in rats treated with cocaine has recently been found to be persistently decreased.[23] Furthermore, hyperprolactinemia[1] and decreased homovanillic acid (HVA)[24] have been reported in human cocaine users and are consistent with functional DA depletion. Hyperprolactinemia and HVA reductions occur several weeks after the cessation of cocaine use, suggesting that DA depletion worsens and persists after stimulant abstinence.

The mechanism of DA depletion by central stimulants has been ascribed to the blockade of DA reuptake from the synapse.[1,3] After reuptake, DA is normally stored in secretory vesicles and reutilized by the presynaptic neuron. The blockade of DA reuptake prevents this "recycling" by trapping DA in the synapse where it is exposed to metabolism. DA depletion would therefore be expected to occur with all agents that block DA reuptake (including amphetamine and methylphenidate), although cocaine has been most studied in this regard.

While the step from neurochemical alterations to clinical symptomatology is always hazardous and speculative, it should not be avoided out of intimidation. Stimulant reward and euphoria have been connected with DA activation. We hypothesized that DA depletion similarly produces stimulant craving.[3,25] One might conceptualize a continuum in which craving and euphoria represent opposite poles, with satiation at the midpoint. The anti-craving efficacy of bromocriptine, a DA receptor agonist, further supports the DA depletion hypothesis of stimulant craving.[25] Since craving is the crucial negative reinforcer of stimulant addiction, its biological basis may serve as an indicator of addictiveness in general. In other words, DA reuptake blockers might, as a class, constitute highly addictive agents based on their ability to stimulate and then deplete pleasure circuitry in the brain.

THERAPEUTIC INDICATIONS OF CENTRAL STIMULANTS

Stimulants have been proposed for a number of therapeutic indications. In the nineteenth century, cocaine was marketed as a health tonic to be used for fatigue, depression, toothache, and even as a pile remedy. Amphetamines were used widely for weight loss, depression and lethargy in the United States, Europe and Asia. The huge quantities of amphetamines manufactured far exceeded their "legitimate" prescriptions as the black market demand for these drugs reflected an insatiable appetite for pleasure center stimulants. Now the major indications for central stimulants are only refractory depression and attention deficit disorder. The most widely prescribed stimulant, methylphenidate, has significant abuse potential. Preclinical studies demonstrate that methylphenidate is self-administered by animals and cannot be discriminated from cocaine or amphetamine.[5] Dextroamphetamine is also prescribed to children for attention deficit disorder. Clinical studies have reported abuse in young patients for whom stimulants have been prescribed,[26] although the notion is unpopular. While therapeutic doses might be below those required to induce euphoria or craving, mood changes do occur with these doses.[27] Careful prospective studies into the potential for subsequent development of addictive illness in children treated with stimulants are lacking.

TREATMENT OF STIMULANT ADDICTION

Stimulant addiction can be classified within the realm of addictive illness, and it responds to the same basic treatment approach. Self-help groups are an effective means of support and education. Behavioral changes should take priority over the attainment of insight. Environmental cues that are capable of provoking craving should be avoided. In particular, friends who use stimulants (or other drugs) should be entirely avoided. Complete abstinence from other addictive substances (including alcohol and marijuana) is crucial. Family education and treatment should be pursued and the patient's lying and manipulative behavior must be replaced with honesty, openmindedness and self-disclosure. Addicts must accept their lack of control over the drug and the disease concept of addiction. Psychological techniques to reduce craving, which are richly embedded in the self-help group philosophy, should be learned and utilized.

Pharmacological approaches to addiction have been largely restricted to the treatment of withdrawal syndromes. The agent or related agent of abuse is substituted and gradually weaned, although the use of clonidine for opiate withdrawal is a notable exception.[28] An additional approach has been the blockade or disruption of euphoria with agents such as naltrexone or Antabuse. Since DA depletion was hypothesized to underlie cocaine craving, direct DA agonists such as bromocriptine and amantadine have been administered and found effective as anti-craving agents.[29,30] Bromocriptine rapidly reverses cocaine craving within minutes, supporting the DA depletion hypothesis of stimulant craving. Tricyclic antidepressants may also be effective in cocaine craving after several weeks.[29] Pharmacotherapy should be viewed as an adjunctive treatment within the context of drug rehabilitation and not as treatment in and by itself.

CONCLUSIONS

This chapter has reviewed the addictiveness of central stimulants. Particular emphasis has been placed on the role of pleasure centers, and the dynamic reinforcement of euphoria and craving in stimulant addiction. It is clearly our contention that drug euphoria and drug craving are the predominant forces that drive the cycle of addiction, and the critical factors to be evaluated in the definition of addiction in general. Also characteristic of addiction is the progressive loss of control over the cycle of craving and euphoria, and the tolerance of medical, psychosocial and legal hazards that develop with compulsive drug use.

It may be a human characteristic to resist the notion that machine-like reward centers can influence our behavior and values to the degree seen with severe drug addiction. This prejudice might explain why stimulant addiction, which involves euphoria and craving without a severe withdrawal syndrome, has been minimized. On the other hand, our preoccupation with "physical" symptoms places an overemphasis on the importance of withdrawal syndromes in the perpetuation of addiction and the conceptualization of addictive disorders. We are biased against viewing ourselves as pleasure-seeking and craving-responsive organisms. Once this bias is overcome, we will be left with a much more sensible understanding of addiction, and new avenues to pursue in its treatment.

REFERENCES

1. Dackis CA, Gold MS, Pottash ALC. Central Stimulant Abuse: Neurochemistry and Pharmacotherapy. Adv Alcohol Sub Abuse. 1987; 6(2): 7-21.

2. Wise RA, Bozarth MA. A psychomotor stimulant theory of addiction. Psych Rev. 1987; 94: 469-492.

3. Dackis CA, Gold MS. New concepts in cocaine addiction: The dopamine depletion hypothesis. Neurosci Biobehav Rev. 1985; 9: 469-477.

4. Deneau GA, Yanagita T, Seevers MH. Self-administration of psychoactive substances by the monkey. Psychopharmacol. 1969; 16: 30-48.

5. Colpaert FC, Niemegeers CJE, Jannssen PAJ. Discriminative stimulus properties of cocaine: Neuropharmacological characteristics as derived from stimulus generalization experiments. Pharmacol Biochem & Behav. 1979; 10: 535-546.

6. Dackis CA, Gold MS. Neurotransmitter and neuroendocrine abnormalities associated with cocaine use. Psych Med. 1987; 3: 461-483.

7. Angrist B, Lee HK, Gershon S. The antagonism of amphetamine-induced symptomatology by a neuroleptic. Am J Psychiatry. 1974; 131: 817.

8. Seigel RK. New patterns of cocaine use: Changing doses and routes. NIDA Monograph Ser. 1985; 61: 204-220.

9. Pickens R, Harris WC. Self-administration of d-amphetamine by rats. Psychopharmacol. 1968; 12: 158-163.

10. Dackis CA, Gold MS, Sweeney DR, Byron JP. Single-dose bromocriptine reverses cocaine craving. Psych Res. 1987; 20: 261-264.

11. Post RM, Kopanda RT, Black KE. Progressive effects of cocaine on behavior and central amine metabolism in the rhesus monkey: relationship to kindling and psychosis. Biol Psychiatry. 1976; 11: 403-419.

12. Kilbey MM, Ellinwood EH. Chronic administration of stimulant drugs:

Response modification. In: Kilbey MM, Ellinwood EH, eds. Cocaine and Other Stimulants. New York: Plenum Press, 1977, pp. 419-429.

13. Gawin FH, Kleber HD. Abstinence symptomatology and psychiatric diagnosis in cocaine abusers. Arch Gen Psychiatry. 1986; 43: 107-113.

14. Cregler LL, Mark H. Medical complications of cocaine abuse. N Engl J Med. 1986; 315: 1495-1500.

15. Itkonen J, Schnoll S, Glassroth J. Pulmonary dysfunction in "freebase" cocaine users. Arch Intern Med. 1984; 144: 2195-2197.

16. Isner JM, Estes NAM, Thompson PD, et al. Acute cardiac events temporarily related to cocaine abuse. N Engl J Med. 1986; 315: 1438-43.

17. Ellinwood EH. Amphetamine psychosis. Description of the individuals and process. J Nerv Mental Dis. 1967; 144: 273.

18. Siegel RK. Cocaine hallucinations. Am J Psychiatry. 1978; 135: 309-314.

19. Yokel RA, Wise RA. Increased lever pressing for amphetamine after pimozide in rats: Implications for a dopamine theory of reward. Sci. 1975; 187: 547-549.

20. Roberts DCS, Koob GF, Klonoff P, Fibiger HC. Extinction and recovery of cocaine self-administration following 6-OHDA lesions of the nucleus accumbens. Pharmacol Biochem Behav. 1980; 12: 781-787.

21. Goeders NE, Smith JE. Cortical dopaminergic involvement in cocaine reinforcement. Sci. 1983; 221: 773-775.

22. Taylor D, Ho BT, Fagen JD. Increased dopamine receptor binding in rat brain by repeated cocaine injections. Commun Psychopharmacol. 1979; 3: 137-142.

23. Wyatt RJ, Karoum F, Suddath R, Fawcett R. Persistently decreased brain dopamine levels and cocaine. JAMA. 1988; 259: 2996.

24. Extein I, Potter WZ, Gold MS, Andre P. Rafuls WA, Gross DA. Persistent neurochemical deficit in cocaine abuse. Am Psych Assoc Abstr. 1987; NR 61.

25. Dackis CA, Gold MS. Bromocriptine as a treatment of cocaine abuse. Lancet. 1985; 1: 1151-1152.

26. Goyer P, Davis G, Rappaport J. Abuse of prescribed stimulant medication by a 13-year-old hyperactive boy. J Am Acad Child Psychiatry. 1979; 18: 170-175.

27. Barkley R. A review of stimulant drug research with hyperactive children. J Child Psych Physiol. 1977; 18: 137-165.

28. Gold MS, Pottash ALC, Extein I, et al. Clonidine in acute opiate withdrawal. N Engl J Med. 1980; 302: 1421-1422.

29. Dackis CA, Gold MS. Pharmacological approaches to cocaine addiction. J Sub Abuse Treatment. 1985; 2: 139-145.

30. Tennant FS, Sagherian AA. Double-blind comparison of amantadine hydrochloride and bromocriptine mesylate for ambulatory withdrawal from cocaine dependence. Arch Intern Med. 1987; 147: 109-112.

The Opioids:
Abuse Liability
and Treatments for Dependence

Joseph W. Ternes, PhD
Charles P. O'Brien, MD, PhD

SUMMARY. The opioids vary greatly in addictive potential, from the highly addictive such as heroin to the opioid antagonists such as naltrexone, which can be used to treat opioid dependence and overdose. The various opioid compounds have different euphorigenic properties and also produce withdrawal syndromes of distinct patterns of duration and intensity. Dependence liability is affected by both the pleasure-seeking motives for initiating drug use and the painful consequences of abstinence or withdrawal. Detoxification, which takes 7-10 days for the short-acting opioids, is usually the first stage in treatment. Methadone is often used as a preliminary stage in detoxification, but some patients are maintained on methadone for years, since it allows them to lead relatively normal lives. Non-opioid drugs used to control withdrawal symptoms include clonidine. After detoxification, naltrexone, a long-acting opioid antagonist, can be administered orally to prevent relapse.

INTRODUCTION AND TERMINOLOGY

Opium was the first drug to be recognized as an addiction problem in the United States. During the past hundred years, new opium derivatives (opiates) and opiate-like drugs (opioids) have been developed in an effort to find an effective pain reliever which did not

---

Joseph W. Ternes and Charles P. O'Brien are affiliated with the Department of Psychiatry, University of Pennsylvania School of Medicine, and the Philadelphia VA Medical Center.

27

have a high abuse potential. The efforts to separate analgesic effects from euphoria-producing effects have been largely unsuccessful.

The dependence liability of an agent is determined by a number of factors, including: the drug's ability to produce withdrawal symptoms sufficiently intense to elicit drug-seeking behavior; its ability to suppress withdrawal symptoms caused by abstinence from other opioids; its tendency to produce tolerance with chronic use; and, most importantly, the intensity, degree, and duration of the euphoria induced. Although most opioids are readily absorbed from the gastrointestinal tract, nasal mucosa, and lung, and from subcutaneous or intramuscular injection, those that can be administered intravenously provide the greatest intensity of "rush" or rapid onset of euphoria. Those that most easily cross the blood-brain barrier have the most rapid onset of action and the highest abuse potential.

There are three different types of narcotic analgesics: the natural alkaloids derived from opium such as morphine; the semi-synthetic chemical modifications of morphine such as heroin; and the synthetic agents which bear only subtle similarities to the structure of morphine such as meperidine. These narcotic analgesics are now commonly classified within a larger category, the opioids, which also includes the narcotic antagonists and the endogenous opioid peptides.

ABUSE LIABILITY

The terms abuse, dependence, psychological dependence and addiction have been defined in the introduction to this volume. As noted, there has been considerable confusion over the years in the definition of these terms by various groups. During the early 1980's, the American Psychiatric Association in collaboration with the World Health Organization set up study groups and committees with the goal of achieving useful definitions which fit clinical data. The result was the definition of psychoactive substance dependence which is contained in DSM III Revised.[1] Dependence is defined in behavioral terms and is consistent across drug categories including stimulants drugs such as cocaine. The distinction between abuse and dependence is made on the basis of severity and numbers of specific symptoms. This definition is considered to be an advance over previous versions because of its clarity and because it permits early diagnosis of dependence without totally relying on the phenomena of tolerance and withdrawal symptoms.

Information on the relative abuse liability of different drugs in the opioid category comes largely from clinical experience. Some opioids are sought after more avidly than others. While there are about 500,000 heroin addicts in the United States, there are relatively few propoxyphene addicts despite the less restrictive access to the latter. The data on which Table 1 is based have been accumulated from a variety of sources including the authors' experience over 20 years of treating opioid addicts. The rank order is not meant to be precise and it would not apply to all individuals. Certain patients report preferences for lower ranking drugs. The following sections review representative opioid drugs from the three major classes; agonists, agonist-antagonists and antagonists. Information

Table 1. Opioid Abuse Potential and Dependence Liability

Drug	Abuse Potential	Dependence Liability
heroin	high	high
hydromorphone	high	high
oxycodone	high	high
fentanyl	high	moderate
morphine	moderate	high
methadone	moderate	high
meperidine	moderate	high
codeine	low	moderate
propoxyphine	low	low
levorphanol	low	low
LAAM	low	low
butorphanol	low	low
pentazocine	low	low
buprenorphine	low	low
nalbuphine	low	-
nalorphine	low	-
cyclazocine	low	-
naloxone	-	-
naltrexone	-	-

which affects the relative abuse potential and dependence liability for each drug is included.

OPIOID AGONISTS

Morphine is considered the prototypical narcotic analgesic and the standard against which all other analgesic agents are compared. Morphine's major pharmacological effects are due to its action on the central nervous system (CNS) and on the gastrointestinal (GI) tract. The CNS actions are responsible for analgesia, respiratory depression, cough suppression and behavioral changes. The GI actions are responsible for suppressing diarrhea. Morphine modifies the patient's subjective evaluation of pain rather than elevating the pain threshold itself. Hence, although the pain is still felt, the perception is not as aversive because the anxiety and stress associated with the painful stimulus are markedly reduced. However, tolerance to the analgesic effects of morphine is rapidly acquired with chronic dosing.

The general behavioral effects of morphine depend on whether the patient is experiencing pain. In a laboratory situation in the absence of pain, morphine may produce dysphoria (characterized by nervousness fear, nausea, vomiting and CNS depression) leaving the user mentally and physically lethargic for hours. Morphine injection has a histamine releasing effect which produces itching. Morphine also depresses respiratory centers in the medulla. Large doses reduce breathing rate as well as depth. The cause of death in most cases of overdose is respiratory failure since morphine suppresses the brain's sensitivity to elevated levels of carbon dioxide in the blood. However, tolerance also develops to these respiratory depressant actions.

Morphine is not as lipid-soluble as codeine, methadone, and heroin and therefore does not cross the blood-brain barrier as readily. For this reason its onset of action is not as prompt as that of heroin and it is reported to be generally less desirable than heroin to intravenous drug abusers.

Codeine or methylmorphine is widely used as an analgesic and cough suppressing agent. Its pharmacological profile resembles morphine but the effects are milder. Codeine is less potent than morphine as an analgesic and cough suppressant; it produces less sedation, and tolerance develops less rapidly. Codeine is approximately two-thirds more effective orally than parenterally, both as an analgesic and a respiratory depressant. The greater oral efficacy is due to less first-pass metabolism in the liver. Codeine is far less prone to be abused and is available over the counter (without prescription) in some countries without serious abuse problems. However, drug-seeking behavior is sometimes exhibited by codeine users. Codeine may be abused in combination with other drugs. An example is glutethimide (Doriden), which is sometimes abused in combination with codeine.

Heroin or diacetylmorphine, is a semi-synthetic derivative of morphine which is illegal to manufacture or import to the United States because its beneficial properties are considered to be outweighed by its high potential for abuse. Its very rapid onset of action after intravenous administration probably accounts for its overwhelming appeal to opioid dependent individuals. Heroin crosses the blood-brain barrier more rapidly than morphine and produces greater euphoric effects when given in equivalent doses. It is a very potent analgesic, approximately three times as active as morphine. Once in the brain, heroin is hydrolyzed to morphine almost immediately. Hydromorphone (Dilaudid) and oxymorphone (Numorphan) are potent analgesics which are similar to heroin in potency and which produce morphine-like withdrawal symptoms. Hydromorphone cannot be distinguished from heroin in double-blind comparisons by experienced addicts.

Methadone is an effective analgesic that is efficient by oral administration, has an extended duration of action, suppresses opioid withdrawal symptoms, and tends to show persistent effects with repeated administration. Parenterally administered, the effects are very similar to those of morphine, and its overall abuse potential is comparable to morphine. With oral administration, methadone is effective as a substitute for heroin in the treatment of heroin dependence.

Methadone thus is a good illustration of the importance of route of administration and onset of action as factors in abuse liability. By the oral route, methadone has a relatively slow onset of action. Patients receiving a steady daily oral dose experience little or no euphoria. Analgesic effects persist for 4-6 hours, but blockade of opioid withdrawal symptoms persists for 24-36 hours. While opiate addicts do exhibit some drug seeking behavior for oral methadone, they prefer to inject it if possible. In methadone treatment programs, the drug is administered as a liquid mixed with orange juice to make injection difficult.

Levo-alpha-acetylmethadol (LAAM) is a congener of methadol which was developed as a long acting analgesic. It has been successfully used to replace methadone in preventing the onset of withdrawal symptoms in heroin dependent individuals who wish to be maintained on a drug which need be taken only three times per week. The major advantages of LAAM are its longer duration of action, minimal euphoria and lower dependence liability. Thus while methadone has a lower abuse potential than heroin or morphine, the abuse potential of LAAM appears to be lower still, based on patient reports.

Propoxyphene, one of methadone's four stereoisomers, is a centrally active analgesic agent that is used as an alternative to codeine for the relief of mild to moderate pain. (Its side effects include nausea, sedation, dizziness, skin rashes, and toxic psychoses and if injected severe skin irritation.) It has one-half to two-thirds the potency of codeine given orally. Large oral doses have been reported to produce pleasurable effects and abrupt discontinuation of high doses will cause a mild withdrawal syndrome. It has been abused in several parts of the country. However, since high doses produce toxic psychoses and since it is very irritating when injected, it has a small potential for producing dependence. Propoxyphene is an example of a low potency opioid whose abuse potential is limited by side effects which prevent its being used in high doses.

THE AGONIST-ANTAGONISTS

This group of drugs are analgesic drugs which act as antagonists at the mu receptor but exert agonistic effects at one or more of the other opioid receptors.

Pentazocine (Talwin) is an effective analgesic agent that is a weak antagonist at mu receptors and a powerful agonist at kappa receptors. High doses to morphine-dependent subjects precipitate withdrawal symptoms through antagonistic action at the mu receptors. Physical dependence develops with chronic use. The withdrawal syndrome, although milder in intensity, resembles morphine withdrawal in producing abdominal cramps, anxiety, chills, hyperthermia, vomiting, tearing, and sweating. It is also associated with drug-seeking behavior. Pentazocine abuse will sometimes occur if it is injected but not when taken orally. Pentazocine is an example of a drug which was predicted to have a low abuse potential based on pre-marketing human and animal research which demonstrated the above facts about its opioid profile. Nonetheless, pentazocine abuse became a significant public health problem in many parts of the country because street users learned that it could be mixed with other drugs, usually an anti-histamine to provide a reliable "high." Since street heroin in the United States is so diluted with adulterants, even a weak agonist such as pentazocine may be preferred by abusers because the effects, though mild, are consistent. Pentazocine abuse was also seen among chronic pain patients who were allowed to self-administer the drug in a relatively un-supervised fashion in the early 1970's before the abuse potential of pentazocine became widely know.

Buprenorphine, a semi-synthetic opioid derived from thebaine, is a congener of etorphine (a strong agonist) and diprenorphine (an opioid antagonist). It is reported[2] to be equivalent to naltrexone in antagonistic potency and in its duration of narcotic blockade. It resembles methadone in its positive subjective effects but without the severe and protracted withdrawal symptoms. Buprenorphine produces only minimal physical dependence. It is probably safer than the strong opioid agonists since the antagonistic effects tend to prevent lethal respiratory depression even at doses that would otherwise be considered fatal. Some of its subjective and respiratory-depressant qualities are similar to those of morphine but slower in onset and longer lasting. Chronic administration produces morphine-like effects, but naloxone does not precipitate withdrawal symptoms. Abstinence results in a mild withdrawal syndrome that is delayed in onset. Overall, its abuse potential is less than that of morphine.

Buprenorphine has many of the attributes of an excellent treatment for heroin dependence. It will significantly suppress opioid self-administration in heroin addicts, antagonize the effects of injected opioids and it will prevent withdrawal in opioid dependent patients. Thus buprenorphine combines some of the qualities of both methadone and naltrexone. However, the abuse potential of a drug depends in part on its context, the comparable drugs available in the environment. During the late 1980's, buprenorphine has become a drug of abuse in some European countries. In these countries, buprenorphine is available on the black market and it is the subject of considerable drug-seeking behavior, yet in other countries, buprenorphine is uncontrolled.

Butorphanol (Stadol) is a synthetic agonist-antagonist analgesic which neither relieves withdrawal symptoms nor produces withdrawal syndrome in morphine dependent monkeys. Chronic administration produces tolerance and physical dependence. A moderate withdrawal syndrome which resembled cyclazocine withdrawal but with little or no drug-seeking behavior was elicited by the abrupt cessation of chronic dosing in both monkeys and humans. There have been no case reports of overdose deaths and few cases of abuse.[3]

Meptazinol is a mixed agonist-antagonist which is a relatively potent analgesic with faster onset but shorter duration of effect than morphine. Meptazinol precipitates withdrawal signs in morphine dependent monkeys but, like other agonist-antagonists, the physical dependence produced is qualitatively different from that of morphine with milder withdrawal symptoms and less drug seeking behavior. It produces less respiratory depression, constipation and meiosis than other agonist-antagonists such as pentazocine. Negative side effects include drowsiness and dizziness. Meptazinol's abuse potential appears to be less than that of the strong opioid agonists.[4]

Nalbuphine is a partial agonist with powerful antagonist action on the mu receptor. It is less likely to produce dysphoric side effects than pentazocine. It is an effective analgesic, like morphine. It also produces respiratory depression but there is a ceiling on this effect. It has been reported to produce morphine-like euphoria as well as headaches, irritability, and depression. Some subjects develop tolerance and will show drug-seeking behavior after a naloxone-precipitated withdrawal. In abuse potential for nondependent individuals it is similar to pentazocine, i.e., lower than morphine. For those who are morphine-dependent it is still lower in abuse potential because of its potent antagonistic action at the mu receptor.[5]

OPIOID ANTAGONISTS

Naloxone is an opioid antagonist which ordinarily produces few effects unless an opioid agonist has been previously administered. Naltrexone (Trexan) combines the long duration blockading properties of cyclazocine with the pure antagonist effects of naloxone. Both naloxone and naltrexone have clinical effects when the endogenous opioid system has been activated, as in shock or under certain forms of stress. The antagonists are useful in the treatment of opioid overdose cases, and also have therapeutic value in the treatment of highly motivated, drug-free, detoxified opioid addicts. Even after prolonged doses of naloxone or naltrexone, discontinuation does not produce a withdrawal syndrome or drug-seeking behavior. These drugs do not produce analgesia, respiratory depression, sedation or changes in pupil size. They usually cause no gross behavioral effects in nondependent individuals nor do they produce euphoria. Thus, naltrexone and naloxone have no known potential for abuse.

PHARMACOLOGICAL ASPECTS OF OPIOID DEPENDENCE

Chronic use of these drugs produces physiological modifications of the organism which is described as physical dependence. Its development is usually accompanied by the acquisition of drug tolerance. The development of tolerance may contribute to the degree of dependence since the higher the maintenance dose of opioid, the more severe the withdrawal discomfort associated with the withdrawal syndrome. Additionally, the euphorigenic effects which opioids produce in non-tolerant individuals are generally reduced or eliminated as tolerance develops. The memory of the euphorigenic properties of opioids appears to be one of the major factors underlying their high potential for abuse. However, euphoria in an opioid tolerant individual is only obtainable by vastly increasing the dose.

Therefore avoidance of withdrawal pain, which begins sooner and with increased intensity when higher doses of the drug are necessitated by tolerance, probably provides an equally powerful motive for opioid abuse.

Chronic self-administration of opioids frequently results in both tolerance and physical dependence. Although the two are positively correlated, evidence for a causal relationship is equivocal. The question of whether a common mechanism underlies these two phenomena is also unresolved. The analysis of tolerance is potentially important for understanding opioid dependence, even though it is not clear whether tolerance actually causes dependence or directly increases drug self-administration. The assumption that tolerance leads to dependence and increased drug-seeking and self-administration is widely held.

The opioid withdrawal syndrome is a complex set of signs and symptoms occurring after chronic administration of an opioid agonist when that opioid is stopped or a competitive opioid antagonist is administered. The withdrawal syndrome develops over time, with different symptoms developing and reaching peak intensity at different times. The different opioid compounds can produce syndromes with distinct patterns of duration and intensity, and the addictive potential of a given drug depends in part on the severity of the syndrome. The syndrome's severity is also affected by the doses used, frequency of re-dosing, and the length of chronic use. With heroin, meperidine, methadone, and dihydromorphine in particular, there appears to be a direct relationship between the opioid dose and the severity of the withdrawal syndrome.

Syndromes resulting from abstinence are known as natural withdrawal, whereas those induced by administration of antagonist are termed precipitated withdrawal. In general, all of the signs and symptoms seen in natural withdrawal occur in precipitated withdrawal, along with other effects such as weight loss, hypothermia, ptosis, and ejaculation in males. With higher doses of a chronically administered opioid, the effective dose of antagonist required to precipitate withdrawal in 50% of the population (the ED50) decreases proportionally, or, in other words, the effectiveness of a given dose of antagonist increases. Increases in duration of opioid exposure also decrease the ED50 of antagonist needed to precipitate withdrawal. With increased length of exposure, the frequencies of the withdrawal signs change, with some reaching peak or asymptomatic levels prior to others. The pattern of change appears to vary with the dose and the specific agonist. Additionally, more withdrawal symptoms occur as length of chronic exposure increases. Route of administration indirectly influences the severity of withdrawal by determining the level of drug in body tissue over time. Thus, routes of administration such as subcutaneous depot injection that provide relatively constant exposure to the opioid may increase the severity of the withdrawal syndrome.[6]

CONDITIONED TOLERANCE

The processes leading to the acquisition of drug tolerance appear to be parallel, if not identical, to the processes that condition changes in behavior, as both involve adaptive, reversible change in response to stimulation.[7] The parallel is strengthened by the fact that physiologic or pharmacologic treatments that modulate tolerance also affect learning. Although indirect, the evidence suggests that tolerance may be mediated by learning processes. The research has been conducted mainly in animals and will not be discussed here. It has recently been reviewed by Goodie and Demellweek.[8]

CONDITIONED WITHDRAWAL

Not all abused opioids produce withdrawal reactions. Even the frequently abused opioids that are known to produce severe withdrawal syndromes are sometimes taken so infrequently that the conditions for the occurrence of the syndrome are not met. On the other hand, former intravenous opioid addicts frequently relapse even after long drug-free periods. These and other observations concerning human opioid addiction make it clear that elucidating the withdrawal syndrome will provide only a partial description of the mechanisms of opioid addiction.

Pharmacologic approaches have emphasized properties of the opioids to explain dependence, such as the fact that the development of tolerance leads to increases in doses that in turn exacerbate the withdrawal symptoms that result from abstinence. According to this line of thinking, the major reason for continued drug seeking and use is to avoid or escape the pain resulting from opioid abstinence. However, opioid dependence cannot be adequately characterized solely on this pharmacologic basis because tolerance and withdrawal syndromes are themselves the consequences of chronic use. The motives for initiating drug use, such as the desire for euphoric experience, must also be taken into account.

Another approach has attempted to identify aspects of the abuser's personality which may benefit from drug use, such as the need to reduce anxiety or alleviate depression. However, the "addiction-prone personality," although an intuitively attractive notion, has not as yet been identified and assessed independently of the behavior it purports to explain. It thus yields little in terms of added explanatory power beyond current behavioral notions of dependence.

In recent years, it has become increasingly apparent that the development of opioid dependence involves both pharmacologic factors such as tolerance and withdrawal syndromes and behavioral processes such as operant and Pavlovian conditioning. Behavioral pharmacology has evolved as an interdisciplinary field for investigating the effects of drugs on a variety of conditioned and unconditioned behavioral responses. Initially, in experiments involving operant conditioning, drug effects were typically demonstrated by observing how stable baseline behavior changes with drug administration. Other approaches involve reinforcing operant behavior with drug administration in order to study how a given drug can influence behavior by exerting reinforcing, aversive, or discriminative effects. In Pavlovian conditioning experiments, drugs have been shown to be able to serve as either conditional or unconditional stimuli. Repeated administration sets in motion the Pavlovian conditioning process, which will then influence or enhance chronic drug effects (conditioned drug effects), and which may also elicit responses opposing the drug effects (conditioned tolerance). Thus the drug appears to control the reinforcement contingency. Henningfield, Lucas, and Bigelow[9] have surveyed clinical investigations dealing with the establishment, maintenance, and elimination of drug-related behavior in which they compare different types of drugs and findings of both human and animal studies. Although dependence can result solely from repeated administration, it is clear that behavior variables can greatly influence the degree of dependence experienced. O'Brien, Ehrman, and Ternes[10] have described classical conditioning studies in human subjects that focus on the conditioning of opioid withdrawal symptoms and on the results of incorporating conditioning principles in treatment programs. Schuster[11] provides a broad-ranging discussion of how behavioral work has influenced treatment approaches and the possibilities for future advances in this area.

Opioid dependence and withdrawal are usually studied by measuring changes in behavior-dependent variables, many of which appear to be functions of the pharmacologic condition of the organism, and this aspect of dependence has not yet been well studied. Although dependence has been well characterized in terms of respondent or physiologic effects, the problem of addiction in humans involves more complex behavioral and sociological variables. Only a few complex behavioral phenomena have been studied in the laboratory, and systematic study of the effects of pharmacologic variables on these behaviors has been infrequent. In one such study of conditioned withdrawal in the rat, Wikler[12] suggested that behavioral phenomena associated with opioid dependence may be dissociated from the pharmacologic state of the organism. These and other data suggest that conditioned drug behaviors are probably determined by a large number of variables and that behavioral changes associated with opioid dependence are not as closely related to pharmacologic condition as are the unconditioned respondent behaviors. Opioid dependence is a complex phenomenon involving many interrelated behavioral responses that ultimately requires behavioral approaches for successful treatment.

TREATMENT MODALITIES

Because opioid abusers suffer from a complex of medical and social problems, multiple treatment approaches are usually indicated. In some cases, for example, behavior therapy or psychotherapy might be used in conjunction with methadone maintenance or residential treatment in a drug-free therapeutic community.

Detoxification

In its simplest form, detoxification simply means withdrawal of the drug on which the patient is dependent. Detoxification and the resulting withdrawal syndrome are usually quite uncomfortable, because a dependent individual has adapted to the presence of the externally supplied opioid. Normal functioning then requires the presence of the drug. To ease the discomfort of the withdrawal syndrome, one can give gradually decreasing doses of either the opioid on which the patient is dependent or another opioid. Any drug in the opiate category can suppress the opiate withdrawal syndrome, but drugs that are short-acting or not active when given by mouth are not practical for detoxification. A drug commonly used for detoxification is methadone. It blocks withdrawal for 24-36 hours and it is quite active when given orally. A typical street heroin addict can start with 20 to 30 mg of methadone and decrease to zero in 7-10 days.

While detoxification from short-acting opioids takes only 7-10 days, mild withdrawal symptoms may persist for months thereafter. Protracted withdrawal is a significant problem for individuals detoxifying from long-acting opioids such as methadone, and perhaps also for those withdrawing from shorter-acting opioids when these have been abused over a long period of time. General clinical experience suggests that very gradual detoxification results in less discomfort, longer retention in drug-free treatment, and, by implication, improved outcomes.

Usually, detoxification is only the first step in a longer-term treatment plan. Since detoxification reduces drug dependency, thus breaking the pattern of addictive behavior and alleviating the financial strain of maintaining an expensive habit, detoxification may be viewed as an end in itself by some patients. In any case, it does provide an opportunity for the patient to proceed to longer-term treatment and relapse prevention programs. Simpson and Sells[13] reported a decline of 33% in daily opioid use by the end of one year following detoxification, and a 66% decline at three-year follow-up.

Methadone Maintenance

Since its legalization as a treatment for heroin addiction in the 1960s, methadone has proved valuable in maintaining patients who either are unable to detoxify or relapse shortly after detoxification. Currently about 80,000 patients are being treated by methadone in more than 500 programs throughout the U.S. In general, patients on oral methadone either reduce or eliminate use of illegal opioids. Unlike naltrexone, methadone is fairly well accepted by most patients, allowing them to engage in social and occupational rehabilitation, and reducing criminal activity motivated by the high cost of maintaining a drug habit. Although methadone stabilization is frequently viewed as a preliminary stage for detoxification and transfer to drug-free treatment, some patients remain on methadone maintenance for many years, since it enables them to lead relatively normal lives. Kreek[14] studied long-term cases and found no evidence of toxic effects from long-term methadone maintenance.

Originally, methadone was used at relatively high doses that blocked or blunted euphoric effects of other drugs. However, these doses can produce sedation and some euphoria. Dose should be adjusted so that the patient has no symptoms of withdrawal and no urges for additional opiate drugs. There is a tendency in current practice to utilize low doses of methadone in an effort to avoid producing additional dependence. However the dose must be high enough to produce cross tolerance to opioid drugs obtained on the street. The proper use of methadone involves regular monitoring of urine to determine whether additional drugs are being taken by the patient, appropriate dose adjustments, and counseling or psychotherapy to help the patient with their overall rehabilitation.

The question always arises concerning length of time that a patient should be on methadone. Some patients wish to remain in treatment for years because they are able to function normally on the drug and they have failed numerous prior attempts to remain totally drug free. Others who wish to detoxify and who have obtained employment and a stable life style are able to gradually withdraw from methadone. Stimmel et al[15] found that 57% of such patients remained drug-free at follow-up 31 months later. However, such patients constitute a small minority of the population usually seen in methadone treatment programs. In general, the best outcomes are produced by programs that also employ behavioral approaches, such as contingency contracting along with methadone.

Mixed Agonists-Antagonists

Although it was once thought that any drug that reversed morphine withdrawal would produce comparable dependence, it was later discovered that not all drugs with opioid agonist effects produce opioid-type dependence in humans. Martin and Gordetsky[16] showed that nalorphine's withdrawal syndrome is qualitatively different from that associated with morphine. More recently, cyclazocine withdrawal has been found to differ significantly from that of morphine. These observations led to the discovery of the multiple opioid receptor types already discussed.

Buprenorphine is a mixed agonist-antagonist with potential usefulness as an aid to detoxification. As an antagonist, it is equivalent to naltrexone in potency and duration of narcotic blockade. As an agonist it produces morphine- or methadone-like subjective effects; however, it does not produce the severe and protracted withdrawal symptoms of either drug. Rather, a mild, rather negligible withdrawal syndrome ensues for approximately two weeks following abrupt cessation of buprenorphine maintenance. Thus, it is said to combine in one drug the beneficial qualities of the two leading pharmacotherapies for opioid addiction. Thus far no large scale clinical trials have been attempted and this use of buprenorphine remains experimental.

Non-Opioid Detoxification Aids

Recently, it has been found that some non-opioid drugs are effective in treating opioid withdrawal symptoms. Gold et al.[17] reported that clonidine inhibited naloxone-precipitated withdrawal signs in rats. Katz and Valentino[18] found that in rhesus monkeys, clonidine modifies some but not all signs of opioid withdrawal, whereas morphine modifies a broader spectrum of signs in a dose-dependent manner. Katz concluded that while morphine reverses withdrawal through a mechanism fundamental to complete expression of the syndrome, the mechanism by which clonidine modifies withdrawal is different, involving non-opioid receptors and permitting withdrawal to proceed in the absence of severe withdrawal reactions. Redman[19] has suggested that opioid withdrawal is similar to anxiety reactions and that the signs and symptoms associated with both involve activation of noradrenergic neurons of the locus coeruleus. This hypothesis is based on the similarity of the manifestations of withdrawal and of anxiety, in addition to the fact that both are reversed by clonidine.

Stimulation of endogenous opioids is theoretically an excellent way to treat opiate dependence. Perhaps chronic opioid abuse has suppressed or deranged the endogenous system and thus the patient is prevented from being comfortable in the drug free state. Efforts to stimulate endogenous opioids have included acupuncture and transcutaneous electrical stimulation. While there have been some very interesting case reports, thus far there is no published study showing evidence as to the efficacy of these techniques in a controlled study.

RELAPSE PREVENTION

Naltrexone

After detoxification, naltrexone may prove a useful adjunct in preventing relapse. A long-acting opioid antagonist, naltrexone occupies the opioid receptors and prevents opioids such as heroin from producing their usual effects. After detoxification, a patient can take naltrexone (Trexan) two to three times a week as protection from the rewarding or reinforcing effects of an opioid in the event that the patient impulsively re-doses with an opioid. Used in this way, naltrexone may also be beneficial by providing experiences of active extinction or unrewarded occurrence of the conditioned response that possibly motivated the abortive attempt to return to drug use.

Naltrexone is not addictive, is effective against all opioids, is long-acting, may be administered orally, and has only a few minor side effects at effective doses. However, the drug is not widely accepted in most drug-abusing populations, appealing only to a highly motivated sub-population of patients who wish to avoid any recurrence of opioid-induced euphoria. Naltrexone is the treatment medication of choice for white-collar drug abusers such as physicians, nurses, and others with ready access to opioids.

REFERENCES

1. Diagnostic and Statistical Manual of Mental Disorders, Third Edition, Revised. Washington, D.C.: American Psychiatric Assoc. Press. 1987. 567 pp.

2. Jaffe JH, Martin WR: Opioid analgesics and antagonists. In Gilman AG, Goodman LS, Rall TW, & Murad F. (eds.): The Pharmacological basis of therapeutics (7th ed., pp. 491-531). New York: Macmillan, 1985.

3. Pachter LJ, Evers RP: Butorphanol. Drug and Alcohol Dependence 1985; 14:325-338.

4. Holmes B, Ward A: Meptazinol: A review of its pharmacodynamic and pharmacokinetic properties and Therapeutic efficacy. Drugs 30; 285-312, 1985.

5. Errick JK, Heel RC: Nalkuphine: A preliminary review of its pharmacological properties and therapeutic efficacy. Drugs 1983; 26(3): 191-211.

6. Jaffe JH: Drug addiction and drug abuse. In Gilman AG, Goodman LS, Rall TW, Murad F, (eds.): The pharmacological basis of therapeutics. (7th ed, pp. 532-576), New York: Macmillan, 1985.

7. Dews PB: Behavioral tolerance. In Krasnegor NA, (ed.): Behavioral tolerance: Research and treatment implications. NIDA Research Monograph No. 18 Washington, DC: U.S. Government Printing Office, 1978.

8. Goodie AJ, Demellweek C: Conditioning factors in drug tolerance. In: Golderberg S, Stolerman I (eds.): Behavioral analysis of drug dependence. San Diego: Academic Press, 1986.

9. Henningfield JE, Lucas SE, & Bigalow GE: Human studies of drugs as reinforcers. In: Goldberg S, Stolerman I (eds.): Behavioral analysis of drug dependency. San Diego: Academic Press, 1986.

10. O'Brien CP, Ehrman RN & Ternes JW: Classical conditioning in human opioid dependence, In: Goldberg S, Stolerman I, (eds.): Behavioral analysis of drug dependence. San Diego: Academic Press, 1986.

11. Schuster CR: Implications of laboratory research for the treatment of drug dependence. In Goldberg S, Stolerman I, (eds.): Behavioral analysis of drug dependence. San Diego: Academic Press, 1986.

12. Wikler A: Conditioning factors in opiate addiction and relapse. In Wilner DI, Kasselbaum GG (eds.): Narcotics. New York: McGraw-Hill, 1965, 85-100.

13. Simpson DD, Sells SB: Effectiveness of treatment for drug abuse: An overview of the DARP Research Program. Advances in Alcohol and Substance Abuse, 1982; 2:7-29.

14. Kreek MJ: Medical complications in methadone patients Ann. NY Acad. Sci. 1978; 311:110-134.

15. Stimmel B, Goldberg J: Ability to remain abstinent after methadone detoxification JAMA 1977; 237:1216-1220.

16. Martin WR, Gordetsky CW: Demonstration of tolerance to and physical dependence on N-allylnormorphine (Nalorphine). J. Pharmacol. Exp. Ther. 1965; 150:437-442.

17. Gold MS, Redman DE, Kleber HD: Clonidine in opiate withdrawal. Lancet 1978; 1:929-930.

18. Katz JL, Valentino RJ: The opiate quasiwithdrawal syndrome in the rhesus monkey: Comparisons of effects of cholinergic agents and naloxone precipitated withdrawal. Psychopharmacology 1984; 84:12-15.

19. Redman DE, Jr: Clonidine and the primate locus ceruleus: Evidence suggesting anxiolytic and anti-withdrawal effects. In Lal H, Fielding S, (eds.): Psychopharmacology of clonidine. New York: Alan R Liss, 1981.

Alcohol: Mechanisms of Addiction and Reinforcement

Michael J. Lewis, PhD

SUMMARY. This chapter examines positive and negative reinforcement mechanisms which play a significant role in alcohol abuse and alcoholism. Consideration is given to the role of euphoria and anxiolytic effects of alcohol as the basis of positive reinforcement, and physical dependence and aversive consequence of drinking as the basis of negative reinforcement. The motivational significance of each of these is discussed with respect to various animal models of addiction and clinical and human research. Brain neurochemistry, neuropharmacology and genetic research data are evaluated from the perspective of reinforcement mechanisms involved with alcohol addiction.

INTRODUCTION

Ethyl alcohol (ethanol) is a psychoactive drug found in alcoholic beverages. Chronic consumption of excessive amounts of these beverages leads to alcohol addiction. While these facts are not surprising to many, the information is not known to all. Recently, the Federal government in considering the issue of warning labels on alcoholic beverages determined that there was a need to state both facts as key messages to be used in these labels.

Michael J. Lewis is affiliated with the Department of Psychology, Howard University, Washington, DC 20059. Correspondence may be addressed to the author at the above address. Dr. Lewis is also affiliated with the Office on Scientific Affairs, National Institute on Alcohol Abuse and Alcoholism.

47

Two important criteria in the definition of addiction are tolerance and physical dependence which are produced with chronic heavy drinking. Tolerance develops to many of the physiological and psychomotor effects of alcohol. Most of the behavioral effects of alcohol also show tolerance, although it is unclear whether tolerance develops to the reinforcing effects of alcohol. Physical dependence on, or withdrawal from alcohol can be quite severe and even life-threatening to those severely dependent on alcohol. Table 1 (1) lists the major symptoms of physical dependence. The onset of these symptoms usually occurs with the elimination of alcohol. "Hang-over" and insomnia appear first followed by agitation, anorexia, tremor and anxiety. The later phase of withdrawal involves more severe reactions. Fatalities may occur in 10% of those untreated for withdrawal.

Alcohol use and abuse is certainly among the highest of all drugs affecting broad segments of the population. Many individuals find consumption of alcoholic beverages pleasant. These pleasant effects reinforce alcohol-seeking and are important factors in alcohol abuse and alcoholism. While there is some consensus about the role of the pleasant "effect" that alcohol produces, the nature of the effect remains an open question. There is considerable disagreement as to whether alcohol produces positive reinforcement or reward by generating euphoria or by producing another affective state, anxiety reduction. Another common hypothesis is that alcohol reward may be acquired through its association with pleasant social situations (e.g., drinking with friends or at parties). While all

Table I. Alcohol Withdrawal Syndrome

Major clinical components	Early or minor dependency	Late or major dependency or delirium tremens
Symptoms or signs	Mild agitation	Extreme overactivity (speech,
	Anxiety	psychomotor, autonomic)
	Restlessness	Disorientation
	Tremor	Confusion
	Anorexia	Disordered sensory perception
	Insomnia	
Latency Postethanol	0-48 hr	24-150 hr
Peak of effect	24-36 hr	72-96 hr
Severity	Mild	Potentially life-threatening
Seizures	Yes, 6-48 hr	No

of these hypotheses are possible, it may well be that alcohol's rewarding effects are a combination of these and perhaps other factors.

As will be apparent in the following review of alcohol addiction, much of the research has focused on the rewarding effects which alcohol produces. Another aspect of the addiction, however, may be the role played by aversive consequences of excessive and chronic alcohol consumption. In this chapter, consideration will be given to the possibility that in addition to rewarding effects, these aversive consequences may be absent or of less motivational significance to the alcoholic or alcohol abuser.

BASIC RESEARCH FINDINGS

Investigation of the reinforcing effects of alcohol have included studies of oral consumption, intravenous self-administration and brain stimulation reward in laboratory animals. All have provided valuable information about the mechanisms which mediate the reinforcing effects of alcohol as they have for other drugs of abuse.

Studies of Oral Consumption

Simple consumption of and operant responding for alcohol solutions have been employed by many researchers to demonstrate its rewarding properties. Several excellent reviews have been published on this research (2,3). They point out that the aversive taste properties and possible peripheral post-ingestional consequences have required food or water deprivation to induce and maintain consumption in animals of random genetic stock. After frequent exposure to alcohol, animals are usually tested under ad libitum food and water conditions. The strength of alcohol's rewarding properties is usually evaluated by preference of alcohol over water.

The use of alcohol solutions sweetened by either sucrose (4) or saccharin (Koob, personal communication) has also been found to produce high levels of initial consumption in undeprived animals. Employing a "sucrose fading" technique where the amounts of the sweetener are slowly reduced, alcohol consumption has been shown to remain high and to function as reward for operant responding (5). With such procedures, rats consume high concentrations of ethanol which produce intoxication, high blood alcohol concentrations, and physical dependence. Rats will learn to even consume very high alcohol concentrations which are usually aversive (e.g., 40% v/v or more; (6). Under such conditions, it is assumed that the animals are administering alcohol for its pharmacological properties and not because of conditioned secondary reinforcement or other effects. The establishment of physical dependence has generally not been found to either motivate oral self-administration or to enhance the behavior in animals already self-administering ethanol (7,8).

Intravenous Self-Administration

Direct intravenous alcohol has also been found to reward operant behavior in both rats (10) and monkeys (11). With this procedure, as with oral self-administration, the apparent initial subjective effects make it difficult to induce administration of alcohol to randomly bred animals. Animals are frequently first trained to lever-press for other reinforcing drugs such as morphine or cocaine (11). Once stable and reliable performance for these drugs is established, then alcohol is substituted for them. Stable responding can be maintained for alcohol alone for considerable periods of time with blood alcohol concentrations sufficient to induce intoxication and physical dependence. The failure of alcohol alone to function as a reward in this self-administration paradigm has cast some doubt about alcohol's intrinsic rewarding properties. As with oral self-administration, physical dependence does not seem to enhance alcohol reinforcement with intravenous self-injection (8). Moreover, dependent animals performing under this paradigm will voluntarily and spontaneously terminate self-administration thereby initiating withdrawal.

Electrical Brain Stimulation Reward

Electrical stimulation of specific brain sites has been found to function as a positive reinforcer for a variety of behaviors (12). This brain stimulation reward (BSR) or self-stimulation (as it is also known) has been used to evaluate many drugs of abuse. Extensive research on opioids, amphetamine and cocaine indicates that these compounds increase response rate and/or lower BSR threshold (for review see notes 13,14). These effects reflect a summation of the rewarding properties of the brain stimulation. BSR is widely considered an animal model of the "high" or euphoria produced by drugs and together with self-administration, they are the two principal experimental models of substance abuse.

Previous research on the effects of alcohol on BSR have been variable and often conflicting (for review see note 15). Several researchers have found that alcohol fails to reliably facilitate BSR rate of response, as distinct from other substances of abuse. Some report that at low doses, facilitation occurs at some sites within the lateral hypothalamus-medial forebrain bundle (LH-MFB) area, but this may vary from animal to animal (16).

Generally, sites elsewhere have not been thoroughly investigated. Recent reports (17) have found more consistent facilitatory effects of alcohol when measures other than response rate were used to determine reward. Research (18) employing BSR threshold (a measure of the amount or frequency of rewarding electrical current applied to the brain) has shown that alcohol reliably lowers BSR threshold at LH-MFB sites at low to moderate doses (see Figure 1). This facilitation was not found in posterior ventral tegmental (VT) brain sites where alcohol had no effect at several low to moderate doses. High doses of alcohol generally interfered with responding at all sites and threshold was increased. Rate of response which was also concurrently measured in these studies proved to be much more variable at all doses and brain sites. These data suggest that there may be specificity with respect to brain sites which mediate alcohol reward. The possibility is further suggested by data that the opioid antagonist naloxone has no effect on LH BSR, but disrupts BSR at VT sites (19). This is the exact opposite of the effects that alcohol produces and suggests that there are differential brain sites mediating alcohol and opioid reward.

Route of administration of alcohol and time of testing may be important variables to consider in evaluating alcohol effects on BSR. Recently, Kornetsky (20) has found that his own generally

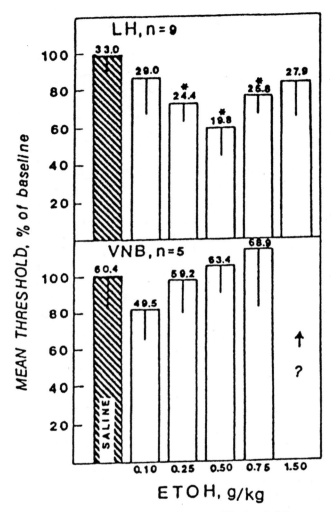

FIGURE 1. Effects of five doses of ethanol on BSR threshold expressed as the percentage of baseline. Numbers above each bar are absolute threshold values in microamperes. Vertical lines within each bar are the S.E.M. Asterisks indicate significant differences from baseline ($p < 0.05$) (Lewis and June, 1990).

negative results with studies of alcohol effects on BSR seem to be a function of whether the alcohol is intraperitoneally injected by the experimenter or is self-administered by the experimental animal. Using oral self-administration of alcohol, Kornetsky found that alcohol increased BSR response rate (20). He is currently investigating the effects of this route of administration on BSR threshold. The slower absorption of alcohol via the oral route may permit a wider window through which to look for the strong rewarding effects of alcohol which may have been missed when testing sessions are long. Recent data from Lewis (21) show that the threshold lowering effects of alcohol are most reliably seen during the ascending limb of the blood alcohol curve (BAC).

Further investigations of alcohol's effects on BSR threshold at multiple brain sites (particularly by those for which specific neurochemical and physiological characteristics are known) will provide invaluable information about the brain mechanisms which mediate alcohol reward and perhaps the "affective" basis of that reward.

Genetic Preferences for Alcohol

The large individual variation in extent to which initial alcohol exposure seems to function as a reward may result from genetic variability among individuals. Large genetic differences have been found among various rodent strains. For example, non-deprived C57BL/6 mice show high preference for alcohol solutions while BALB/c and DBA/2 mice avoid alcohol. Selective breeding of mice (22) and rats (23) has produced lines which show high levels of oral consumption of ethanol. The selectively bred P (preferring) rats have been found to prefer alcohol at concentrations greater than 30% over water in a two-bottle choice paradigm (24). The P animals will drink to intoxication, perform operant responses for oral and intragastric alcohol and show high blood alcohol concentration (23). The NP (non-preferring) rats, on the other hand, prefer water at all but the lowest concentrations of alcohol.

These data strongly indicate that the alcohol preference is based upon the post-ingestive presumably reinforcing effects of alcohol. However, it is not clear whether the genetic contributions are with regard to increased reward effects in the P rats or decreased oversize consequences of alcohol intake in them. The failure of alcohol to produce aversive signs of intoxication or other aversive post-ingestive responses in P rats may account for increased alcohol preference. Conversely, increased oversize responses in NP rats may account for their decided lack of preference for alcohol. Continued investigation of behavior and brain systems in these two important genetic lines hopefully will provide answers to these questions. These investigators have recently selected new lines of alcohol preferring and non-preferring rats: HAD (high alcohol drinking) and LAD (low alcohol drinking), respectively (Li, personal communication). These new animals were derived from a genetically heterogeneous stock employing essentially the same selection procedures as were employed in deriving P and NP lines. Comparison of brain behavior mechanisms of the two selected preference lines should further provide a better understanding of genetic factors in alcohol reinforcement, both positive and negative.

Drug Interactions with Alcohol Reinforcement and Brain Neurochemistry

Several studies have examined the effects of other drugs of abuse on alcohol reinforcement. Administration of some of these drugs prior to access to alcohol has produced increased alcohol consumption suggesting possible interactions between brain systems mediating alcohol and other drug reward. Opioids, for example, have been found to increase consumption of sweetened alcohol solutions. Morphine and diprenorphine (a mixedagonist/antagonist) have been shown to enhance consumption of sweetened alcohol solutions over water (25). These data suggest a possible linkage between opioid and alcohol reinforcement.

Initial interest was produced by the possibility that condensation of catecholamines with aldehydes may produce opioid-like tetrahydroisoquinolines (TIQ's) within the brain. Similarly, betacarboline alkaloids (BCA) are produced by condensation of serotonin (5-HT) with aldehydes. These compounds could conceivably be produced by excessive alcohol consumption leading to on accumulation of acetaldehyde in the brain. TIQ's continuously infused into the cerebral ventricles of rats have been reported to produce consumption of large quantities of high concentration alcohol over water. These animals exhibited elevated blood alcohol levels, withdrawal, as well as long-lasting preference for alcohol (26). Several more recent reports (27) indicate that intracerebral injections of various TIQ and BCA compounds enhance alcohol consumption. However, considerable controversy exists with this research concerning whether behaviorally significant quantities of them are produced with alcohol consumption.

Inhibiting the synthesis of 5-HT by systemic injection of parachlorophenylalanine (PCPA) decreases alcohol consumption in rats. It is, however, probable that this effect is due to nausea and malaise which PCPA produces that may have elicited a conditioned taste aversion and not due to blockade of 5-HT synthesis. Serotonin depletion, on the other hand, by direct injection of the relatively specific neurotoxin 5,6 dihydroxytryptamine (5,6-DHT), was found to enhance alcohol intake (28). Conversely, 5-HT reuptake blockers (which enhance 5-HT neurotransmission) decrease alcohol consumption in various animal self-administration models (29). Zimelidine, fluvoxamine, fluoxetine, and several other related compounds suppress alcohol consumption in rats. These results have been welcomed by clinicians who have begun extensive clinical investigation of them.

Many researchers believe that dopamine (DA) (30) and perhaps norepinephrine (NE) (31) play a major role in alcohol reward. Antagonism of catecholamine systems, DA and norepinephrine, has generally been found to decrease alcohol consumption. This is generally consistent with the view that they, particularly DA, mediate rewarding events in the brain. Such manipulations are not specific to alcohol reinforcement and have been found with opiate and stimulant reinforcement. Results of some manipulations of catecholamines have been inconsistent. For example, destruction of brain catecholamines by direct injection of the neurotoxin 6-hydroxydopamine into the cerebral ventricles was found to decrease alcohol drinking in some strains of rats, but not in others (28), several findings using specific antagonists of NE synthesis have been found to decrease alcohol drinking (31).

Amphetamine administration also generally decreases alcohol

consumption. This suppression is found over a wide range of amphetamine doses when alcohol consumption occurs in animals that are not food-deprived (30). Under conditions of food deprivation, however, low doses of amphetamine enhanced alcohol consumption over their baseline levels. These investigators (for review see (3)) attempted to determine if both of these effects were due to amphetamine's agonistic effects on brain DA. Pimozide (a DA antagonist) failed to block the suppressant effects of amphetamine, while strongly decreasing alcohol consumption itself. Given the latter finding it was not surprising that the amphetamine-induced increase in alcohol consumption in deprived rats was blocked by pimozide.

The possibility that alcohol reinforcement may involve the benzodiazepine-GABA receptor complex has been raised most recently by reports (32) that the imidazobenzodiazepine inverse agonist R015-4513 blocks the intoxicating and anxiolytic effects of alcohol. Recently, however, Samson and his collaborators (33) have found in some preliminary studies that alcohol self-administration was blocked by the inverse agonists R015-4513 and FG7142. Further research in this area is, of course, necessary to clarify this issue and to more directly determine the role, if any, that the GABA and benzodiazepine receptors may play in alcohol reinforcement and other effects.

Summary and Conclusions

Alcohol functions as a strong reinforcer of alcohol-seeking behaviors in experimental animals. Simple oral consumption, operant behavior for oral and intravenous alcohol administration and facilitation of BSR all demonstrate alcohol's reinforcing effects. It seems clear that the reinforcement is primarily a function of the reward properties of alcohol because physical dependence, which would provide the basis for negative reinforcement, does not lead to initiation or maintenance of self-administration. The research on brain neurochemical systems suggests that multiple neurotransmitters (5-HT, DA, GABA) may play a role in alcohol reinforcement. Data on BSR suggest that despite the multiple mediation, there are specific brain sites which mediate alcohol euphoria. Also, euphoria apparently occurs during the ascending limb of the BAC.

CLINICAL INVESTIGATIONS

Biomedical Studies of Alcohol Euphoria

There have been relatively few rigorous studies of alcohol reinforcement in humans. Many reports have been anecdotal or retrospective suggesting conflicting and paradoxical effects of alcohol on mood. Pleasant mood states highlighted by relaxation and a state of well-being are frequently reported; however, mood changes to dysphoria and anxiety are common as drinking continues. Chronic alcohol abusers often experience anxiety and depression with acute intoxication (34). Clearly these varying effects may be a function of multiple factors including drinking history, personality, other psychiatric disorders as well as degree of tolerance and physical dependence. Examining the effects of alcohol during various portions of the BAC has provided a useful way to analyze the varying affective responses. Although it has been hypothesized that alcohol produces different mood states during the ascending phase of the BAC from those at the peak or descending phase, it has been difficult to measure the behavioral sequence and to determine the relationship between physiological processes and mood changes.

Recently, Mendelson, Lukas and colleagues (35,36) have attempted to determine electrophysiological and neuroendocrine correlates of alcohol self-administration in human subjects. Employing innovative techniques, they have concurrently measured BAC, EEG and plasma adrenocorticotropic hormone (ACTH) and cortisol in subjects who were able to report their subjective mood state using a hand-held manipulanda. Mood and EEG activity were highly correlated with BAC (see Figure 2). Alpha EEG activity generally increased during the ascending limb and was most prominent when subjects reported intense pleasure or euphoria. It returned to baseline during the descending limb of the BAC. Theta activity on the other hand generally increased during the entire two-hour period of measurement. In another study (36), increased plasma ACTH as

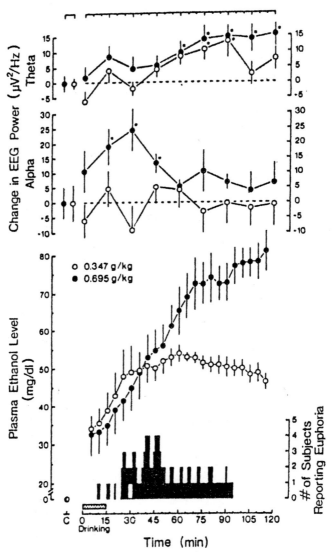

FIGURE 2. Time course of changes in theta (4-8Hz) and alpha (8-13Hz) EEG activity, plasma ethanol levels and reported episodes of euphoria after low dose (o) and high dose (•) ethanol administration. Values represent means ± SEM for six subjects except for the reported episodes of euphoria which are plotted as actual events. The single episode produced by low dose ethanol is indicated by the small white block at 30-31 min. (From Lukas *et al.*: EEG alpha activity increases during transient episodes of ethanol-induced euphoria. *Pharmacol Biochem Behav* 25:889-895, 1986).

well as alpha EEG activity were correlated with episodes of euphoria. These episodes began with 10 minutes of drinking and continued periodically for another 40 minutes and corresponded with relatively low ascending BAC. The percentage of subjects reporting euphoria reached a peak at about 30 minutes after alcohol consumption as did plasma ACTH and alpha EEG activity.

These data were obtained from adult male social drinkers. The positive early effects of alcohol were transient and probably dose dependent. High alcohol doses and chronic abuse have been found to be followed by anxiety and many abnormal endocrine and physiological responses (e.g., impaired adrenocortical responses). Consumption of small amounts of alcohol which enhance alpha EEG and ACTH activity may reverse or normalize these deficits in such individuals.

While chronic alcohol abuse and high BAC are associated with chronic adrenocortical activation and dysphoria, the initial effects of low dose alcohol consumption produce short-term adrenocortical activation and euphoria. Lukas and Mendelson (36) speculate that the adrenocortical action may be due to ethanol-induced central stimulation of corticotropin-releasing factor(CRF) or possibly to ACTH or CRF acting on specific brain regions which presumably mediate reward. They speculate that these acute changes with the rising BAC may produce intense sensations which are like the heroin "rush" or cocaine "high."

Physical Dependence and Anxiolytic Effects on Alcohol Abuse

Chronic administration of high doses of alcohol produces physical dependence. As previously mentioned, animal studies of the role of these highly aversive symptoms suggest that these do not play a major role in alcohol self-administration. There is very little objective or systematic information from human or clinical studies on the relationship between withdrawal symptoms and motivation to drink (37). Many patients, however, anecdotally report relapsing after short periods of self-imposed abstinence in order to escape or avoid the discomfort of withdrawal. Treatment of alcohol dependence by benzodiazepines which are cross-dependent with alcohol is consistent with this observation. Open trial studies of chlordiaze-poxide without patient alcoholics show decreased craving and greater abstinence with the medication. In some of those who experienced alcohol craving, it was associated with symptoms similar to alcohol withdrawal and the strength of the craving corresponded somewhat with the recency of alcohol withdrawal-like experiences. However, human alcoholic subjects, like animal subjects, will spontaneously cease alcohol self-administration despite the onset of withdrawal (38). Many have concluded that alcohol withdrawal is neither a sufficient nor necessary condition for initiating or maintaining alcohol abuse (37).

Although reduction of tension and anxiety is frequently reported by sober alcoholics as major desirable consequences of their drinking, they often fail to experience them after drinking (34). This failure is perplexing because animal studies show that alcohol has substantial anxiolytic effects in various conflict tests (e.g., Geller passive avoidance (39,40)). Anxiolytic effects are also reported in non-alcoholic human subjects (41). Although data are sparse, one might speculate that alcohol produces anxiolytic action at low to moderate doses in non-dependent drinkers; however, these reinforcing effects dissipate with the development of tolerance and physical dependence. Considerable further research is needed on this question.

Pharmacotherapy of Alcohol Abuse

Research on the neuropharmacology of alcohol reinforcement has led to the investigation of several drugs which are new in the treatment of alcohol abuse. There are a variety of drugs which have some rather specific neurochemical actions and represent a newer approach to pharmacotherapy than the use of antimetabolic agents such as disulfiram or calcium carbimide. The first of these are the serotonin re-uptake blockers. As previously mentioned, zimelidine, fluvoxamine, fluoxetine as well as other similar compounds reduce alcohol consumption in animals (29). These compounds exhibit great potential as adjuncts to traditional psychotherapy in the treatment of alcohol dependence.

Another drug which is currently being investigated is buspirone, a putative serotonin receptor agonist with potent anxiolytic properties. It has been found to reduce alcohol consumption in monkeys (41) and is currently being investigated in preliminary clinical trials where it is believed to decrease the desire to drink in anxious alcoholics. Buspirone, unlike benzodiazepine anxiolytics, has very low abuse and dependence liabilities. Considerable further research is, of course, needed on this drug.

Opioid antagonists like naloxone and naltrexone have also been found to reduce alcohol consumption in animals (42). These drugs also decrease alcohol consumption in humans (for review see (43)). Clinical trials of these and other opioids are required to determine their efficacy.

Genetic Risk for Alcohol Reinforcement

Considerable recent interest has been generated by studies showing increased risk for alcoholism among relatives of alcoholics. Several lines of research, including studies of twins, adoptees and half-siblings, suggest that sons of alcoholics, in particular, are at risk for alcoholism (for reviews, see (44)). Based on longitudinal studies of Swedish alcoholics, Cloninger (45) has provided evidence of two types of alcoholics which differ in genetic risk for alcoholism, age of onset of alcoholism and personality. The Type 1 alcoholic (also known as Milieu-Limited) is the more common type representing approximately 75% of male alcoholics. The role genetics plays in this type of alcoholism is of a much lower magnitude than the second type of alcoholism. As shown in Table 2, alcohol-related problems begin after age 25 in this group. An important distinguishing feature of this group is that they exhibit frequent guilt and anxiety over their alcohol dependency and tend to be highly dependent on rewards and to avoid aversive events (46).

Type 2 alcoholism (Male-Limited) represents approximately 25% of male alcoholics and has a very strong genetic basis being apparently passed from father to son (45). Alcohol-related problems (Table 1) begin generally before age 25 and are associated with antisocial behaviors such as aggression and some conflict with law enforcement as well as very little guilt or anxiety over alcohol dependency. Such alcoholics exhibit spontaneous alcohol seeking,

Table 2. Distinguishing Characteristics of Two Types of Alcoholism

	Type of alcoholism	
Characteristic features	Type 1	Type 2
Alcohol-related problems		
Usual age of onset (yrs)	After 25	Before 25
Spontaneous alcohol-seeking (inability to abstain)	Infrequent	Frequent
Fighting and arrests when drinking	Infrequent	Frequent
Psychological dependence (loss of control)	Frequent	Infrequent
Guilt and fear about alcohol dependence	Frequent	Infrequent
Personality traits		
Novelty-seeking	Low	High
Harm avoidance	High	Low
Reward dependence	High	Low

After Cloninger, 1987

higher alcohol consumption and high novelty seeking behaviors (46).

Based upon these characterizations, one might expect that alcohol abuse in these two types of alcoholics may be reinforced differently by alcohol. Type 1 alcoholics may find the anxiolytic actions of alcohol quite rewarding and may binge when stress and anxiety levels are quite high. They may also secondarily desire the euphoric properties of alcohol when life-events provide few rewards. Type 2 alcoholics on the other hand may be influenced by the activation during the euphoric actions of alcohol. This group, however, tends to be more active (46) and, therefore, may drink for the depressant effects of alcohol which may "normalize" their level of activity and impulsiveness. These speculations await more intensive research efforts with alcoholic populations, especially sons of alcoholics.

Reinforcement differences between the two groups may also involve the aversive physiological consequences of alcohol. Type 1 alcoholics tend to exhibit binge drinking followed by periods of guilt and anxiety over their drug abuse. These represent aversive *psychological* consequences for their behavior (45). Moreover, one would expect that they are very likely to experience strong hangovers after their binges simply because of the large amount of alcohol consumed during these episodes. These *physiological* consequences would probably motivate long periods of abstinence as an avoidance of the aversive reaction. Type 2 alcoholics drink more frequently and in greater amounts and do not exhibit guilt or anxiety over their alcohol abuse. This suggests that they either do not experience the severe physiological consequences of drinking or do not find them sufficient to motivate avoidance behavior.

These putative differences in positive and negative reinforcement functioning in alcoholics may be one of the manifestations of the genetic differences between alcoholic subtypes and perhaps between alcoholics and non-alcoholics.

Summary and Conclusions

The clinical and human research closely parallels that with animals concerning alcohol reinforcement, genetic variables and pharmacological mechanisms. Alcohol reinforcement seems to be primarily a function of euphoric and anxiolytic effects. Physical dependence apparently plays a relatively minor role in sustaining drinking. Genetic studies suggest that alcohol's various positive and negative reinforcing effects may differentially reinforce alcohol abuse in Type 1 and Type 2 alcoholics.

OVERALL SUMMARY AND CONCLUSIONS

It is clear from both the animal and human research that alcohol self-administration is reinforcing and that it exhibits the same essential behavioral and pharmacological phenomena as other addicting drugs. Tolerance, physical dependence and self-administration all are produced by alcohol and are important elements in the treatment of alcoholism and alcohol abuse. Alcohol, however, is unique in that its actions on the brain are not easily understood given our current state of knowledge. We have not found a specific "receptor" with which this powerful drug interacts. Euphoria, anxiolytic action, tolerance and physical dependence all are produced through various brain systems, apparently through subtle and perhaps indirect actions. Our task in studying them is exceedingly challenging.

There is considerable optimism that the development of research techniques including new genetic approaches will make further advancement possible in the understanding of alcohol addiction.

REFERENCES

1. Naranjo CA, Sellers EM. Clinical assessment and pharmacotherapy of the alcohol withdrawal syndrome. In: Galanter M, ed. Recent developments in alcoholism: 4, 1986:265-281.

2. Meisch RA. The function of schedule-induced polydipsia in establishing ethanol as a positive reinforcer. Pharmacol Rev, 1976; 27:394-402.

3. Samson HH. Initiation of ethanol-maintained behavior: a comparison of animal models and their implication to human drinking. In: Thompson T, Dews PB, Barrett JE. Advances in Behavioral Pharmacology, vol 6. New Jersey: Lawrence Erlbaum Assoc., 1987,221-248.

4. Reid LD, Hunter GA. Morphine and naloxone modulate intake of ethanol. Alcohol, 1984; 1(1):133-137.

5. Samson HH. Oral ethanol self-administration in rats: Models of alcohol-seeking. Alcoholism: Clin. Exp. Res., 1988; 12(5):591-597.

6. Grant KA, Samson HH. Induction and maintenance of ethanol self-administration without food deprivation in the rat. Pharmacology, 1985: 86:475-479.

7. Mello NK. A review of methods to induce alcohol addiction in animals. Pharmacol Biochem Behav, 1973; 1:89-101.

8. Cicero TJ, Smithloff BR. Alcohol oral self-administration in rats: attempts to elicit excessive intake and dependence. In: MM Gross, ed. Alcohol Intoxication and Withdrawal. New York: Plenum Press, 1973:35.

9. Smith SG. Davis WM. Intravenous alcohol self-administration in the rat. Pharmacological Research Communications. 1974;6:394-402.

10. Deneau G, Yanagita T, Seevers MH. Self-administration of psychoactive substances by the monkey. Psychopharmacologia, 1969;16:30-48.

11. Winger G, Woods, JH. Schedules of ethanol reinforcement. Sixth International Congress of Pharmacology, Helsinki, Finland, 1975;20-25.

12. Olds J, Milner P. Positive reinforcement produced by electrical stimulation of septal area and other regions of rat brain. J Comp Physiol Psychol., 1954; 47:419-427.

13. Wise RA, Bozarth MA. Brain reward circuitry: Four circuit elements "wired" in apparent series. Brain Res Bull, 1984; 12:203-208.

14. Kornetsky C, Esposito RU, McLean S, Jacobson JO. Intracranial self-stimulation thresholds: A model for the hedonic effects of drugs of abuse. Arch Gen Psychiat, 1979; 38:289-292.

15. Kornetsky C, Bain GT, Unterwald EM, Lewis MJ. Brain stimulation reward: Effects of ethanol alcoholism. Clin Exper Res. 1988; 12:609-616.

16. St Laurent J, Olds J. Alcohol and brain centers of positive reinforcement.

In: Fox R, ed. Alcoholism Behavioral Research, Therapeutic Approaches. New York: Springer, 1967:85-106.

17. De Witte P, Bada, MF. Self-stimulation and alcohol administered orally or intraperitoneally. Exp. Neurol., 1983; 82:675-682.

18. Lewis MJ, Phelps RW. A multifunctional on-line brain-stimulation system: investigation of alcohol and aging effects. In: Bozarth MA, ed. Methods of assessing the reinforcing properties of drugs. New York: Springer-Verlag, 1987:463-478.

19. Lewis MJ, Andrade JR, Mebane C, Phelps R. Differential effects of ethanol and opiates on BSR threshold. Soc Neurosci Abstr, 1984; 10:960.

20. Bain GT, Kornetsky C. Ethanol oral self-administration and rewarding brain stimulation. Alcohol, in press.

21. Lewis MJ. Alcohol effects on brain stimulation reward: blood alcohol concentration and site specificity. In: Koob GF, Lewis MJ, Paul SM, Meyer RE, ed. New Approaches to the Neuropharmacology of Alcohol, in preparation.

22. McClearn GE, Roger DA. Differences in alcohol preference among inbred strains of mice. Q J Stud Alcohol, 1959; 20:691-695.

23. Li TK, Lumeng L, McBride WJ, Murphy JM. Rodent lines selected for factors affecting alcohol consumption. Alcohol and alcoholism Suppl, 1987; 1: 91-96.

24. Murphy JM, Gatto GJ, McBride WJ, Lumeng L, Li TK. Operant responding for oral ethanol in the alcohol-preferring P and alcohol-nonpreferring NP lines of rats. Alcohol, 1989, in press.

25. Reid LD, Czirr SA, Bensinger CC, Hubbell CL, Volanth AJ. Morphine and diprenorphine together potentiate intake of alcoholic beverages. Alcohol, 1988: 4(3):161-168.

26. Melchoir CL, Myers RD. Preference for alcohol evoked by tetrahydropapaveroline (THP) chronically infused in the cerebral ventricles of the rat. Pharmacology Biochem Behav. 1977: 7:19-35.

27. Airaksinen MM, Mahonen M, Tuomisto P, Peura P, Ericksson CJP. Tetrahydro-B-carbolines: effect of alcohol intake in rats. Pharmac Biochem Behav., 1983; 18:525-529.

28. Melchior CL, Myers RD. Genetic differences in ethanol drinking of the rat following injection of 6-OHDA, 5,6-DHT or 5,7-DHT into the cerebral ventricles. Pharmacal Biochem Behav. 1976; 5:63-72.

29. Lawrin MO, Naranjo CA, Sellers M. Identification and testing of new drugs for modulating alcohol consumption. Psychopharmacol Bull. 1986: 22:1020-1025.

30. Pfeffer AO. Samson HH. Oral ethanol reinforcement: Interactive effects of amphetamine, pimozide and food-restriction. Alcohol Drug Res. 1985; 6: 37-48.

31. Amit Z, Brown ZW. Actions of drugs of abuse on brain reward systems: A reconsideration with specific attention to alcohol. Pharmacology Biochem Behav. 1982; 17:233-238.

32. Suzdak PD, Glowa JR, Crawley JN, Schwartz RD, Skolnick P, Paul SM. A selective imidazobenzodiazepine antagonist of ethanol in the rat. Science. 1986; 234:1243-1247.

33. Samson HH, Haraguchi M, Tolliver GA, Sadeghi KG. Antagonism of ethanol-induced behavior by the benzodiazepine inverse agonists Ro 15-4513 and FG-7142: relationship to sucrosere inforcement. Pharmacology Biochem Behav. 1989, in press.

34. Nathan PE, O'Brien JS, Lowenstein LH. Operant studies of chronic alcoholism: Interaction of alcohol and alcoholics. In: Roach MK, McIsaac WM, Creaven PJ, Biological aspects of alcohol. New York: 1970, 341-370.

35. Lukas SE, Mendelson JH, Benedikt RA, Jones B. EEG alpha activity increases during transient episodes of ethanol-induced euphoria. Pharmacal Biochem Behav. 1986; 25:889-895.

36. Lukas SE, Mendelson JH. Electroencephalographic activity and plasma ACTH during ethanol-induce euphoria. Biol Psychiatry, 1988: 23:141-148

37. Gorelick DA, Wilkins JN. Specific aspects of human alcohol withdrawal. In: Galanter M, ed. Recent developments in alcoholism. 4. New York: Plenum, 1986:283-305.

38. Mello NK. A semantic aspect of alcoholism. In: Cappell HD, LeBlanc AE. eds. Biological and Behavioral Approaches to Drug Dependence. Toronto: Addiction Research Foundation. 1975:73-87.

39. Koob GF, Thatcher-Britton K, Roberts DCS, Bloom FE. Destruction of the locus coeruleus or dorsal noradrenergic bundle does not alter release of punished responding by ethanol and chlordiazepoxide. Physiol Behav. 1984; 33:479-485.

40. Dalterio SL, Wayner MJ, Geller I, Hartmann RJ. Ethanol and diazepam interactions on conflict behavior in rats. Alcohol, 1988; 5(6):471-476.

41. Collins DM, Myers RD. Buspirone attenuates volitional alcohol intake in chronically drinking monkey. Alcohol, 1987: 4:49-56.

42. Sinclair JD. The feasibility of effective psychopharmacological treatments for alcoholism. Br J Addict. 1987; 82:1213-1223.

43. Reid L, Czirr SA, Milano WC, Hubbell CL, Manha NA. Opioids and intake of alcoholic beverages. In: Proceedings of the 1986 International Narcotics Research Conference: National Institute on Drug Abuse: Research Monograph Series. Rockville, MD: Department of Health and Human Services. 1986:359-362.

44. Symposium: The genetics of alcoholism. Begleiter H. ed. Alcoholism: Clinical and Experimental Research. 1988; 12:457-505.

45. Cloninger CR. Neurogenetic adaptive mechanisms in alcoholism. Science (Wash DC). 1987:236:410-416.

46. Cloninger CR, Sigvardsson S, Bohman M. Childhood personality predicts alcohol abuse in young adults. Alcoholism: Clinical and Experimental Research, 1988; 12:494-505.

Abuse Liability of Barbiturates and Other Sedative-Hypnotics

William W. Morgan, PhD

SUMMARY. The principal action of the sedative-hypnotic drugs, of whom the barbiturates are the most widely known and utilized, is to produce drowsiness and promote sleep. At one time these were also the only drugs available to calm seriously anxious or disturbed people. Unfortunately, in addition to their clinical applications these drugs manifest a very high abuse potential. Experienced drug abusers report feelings of well-being and euphoria while under the influence of these drugs. Self-administration experiments conducted in animals have shown that the barbiturates are potent reinforcing agents. In controlled studies in humans, former drug abusers express a preference for barbiturates over benzodiazepines and will "work" to receive barbiturates. Long term consumption of the sedative-hypnotics, particularly barbiturates, leads to dependence characterized by a severe, potentially life-threatening abstinence syndrome following the abrupt withdrawal of the drug. Withdrawal manifestations include delirium and grand mal seizures. Because of the high abuse potential of these drugs, their manufacture and distribution has been greatly curtailed, and for most clinical applications they have been largely replaced by drugs, e.g., the benzodiazepines, which appear to have much less abuse liability.

DRUGS DISCUSSED

The purpose of this chapter is to discuss and evaluate the abuse potential of the sedative-hypnotics, drugs whose principal action is to induce drowsiness and promote sleep (see Table 1). The label, sedative, is in part misleading as it refers to a time when these

William W. Morgan is affiliated with the Department of Cellular and Structural Biology, University of Texas Health Science Center at San Antonio, 7703 Floyd Curl Drive, San Antonio, TX 78284.

67

TABLE I.   Drugs Discussed in Chapter

Barbiturate Sedative - Hypnotics
    (short - acting)   (long - acting)

Amobarbital	Barbital
Methohexital	Phenobarbital
Pentobarbital	
Secobarbital	

Non Barbiturate Sedative - Hypnotics

Ethchlorvymol	Methyprylon
Glutethimide	Methaqualone
Meprobamate	

Benzodiazepines

Clonazepam	Lorazepam
Clorazepate	Medazepam
Diazepam	Midazolam
Flurazepam	Triazolam

agents were the only compounds available to calm anxious or seriously disturbed people.[1] The discussion will center primarily on the barbiturates. This will be the case in part because of the author's greater familiarity with these compounds, but primarily because these particular drugs have been the "test" substances in almost all of the scientifically controlled hypnotics.

The first barbiturate hypnotic, barbital, was introduced in 1903, and in the ensuing decades more than 50 barbiturates were marketed.[1] In addition to their widespread clinical use, the barbiturates were also very popular and dangerous drugs of abuse, and they became major social and physical health problems in the United States. As a result, the stricter regulation of the manufacture and sale of these drugs and their replacement with other pharmacologic agents, e.g., benzodiazepines, with a higher therapeutic index and reportedly a lower abuse potential, have markedly reduced the misuse of these particular sedative-hypnotics. Although they have been largely replaced, the barbiturates still have some use as short-acting hypnotics and as anticonvulsant agents. Phenobarbital, for example, is still one of the most effective and widely used anticonvulsants against tonic-clonic or grand mal seizures.[2] These drugs are also judged to retain legitimate value as sedatives to decrease restlessness in certain serious illnesses in children and to reduce the apprehension associated with minor medical or dental surgical procedures.[1]

The abuse liability of meprobamate will also be reviewed. This drug was introduced in 1955 and is currently approved as an anti-anxiety agent. However, it is still employed as a treatment for insomnia, particularly in geriatric patients in whom it has been reported to be more effective than the benzodiazepines.[1]

Brief mention will be made of other non-barbiturate sedative-hypnotic agents in order to emphasize the dependence-producing potential of this class of drugs. Unfortunately, most of these compounds have never been critically evaluated in order to determine their comparative abuse potential. Of particular note is methaqualone, which, like many of these drugs, was originally introduced in the United States in 1965 as a non-barbiturate with "low abuse potential." Unfortunately, this drug was quickly observed to have remarkable abuse liability[3] and, because of its widespread misuse, was withdrawn from the American market in 1984. However, methaqualone may continue to be available from illegal sources.

Missing is an in depth discussion of the benzodiazepine sedative-hypnotics which will be covered in a separate chapter by Dr. J. Roache.

DEPENDENCE ON SEDATIVE-HYPNOTICS

One of the most serious aspects of the abuse of the sedative-hypnotics is that the prolonged misuse of these drugs leads to the development of physical dependence characterized by a severe, potentially life-threatening abstinence syndrome following their abrupt withdrawal. The next few paragraphs will briefly review the more salient studies which have characterized the major manifestions associated with this abstinence syndrome.

a. Barbiturates

The first scientifically controlled study of the effects of the chronic consumption and subsequent abrupt withdrawal of barbiturates in humans was conducted by Harris Isbell and his coworkers.[4] In their study there were five male subjects, each with a long history of both narcotic and alcohol abuse. Two subjects were treated chronically with secobarbital, two received pentobarbital and one was given amobarbital.

As the daily dosages of these drugs were cautiously increased, the subjects began to manifest increasing signs of moderate to severe intoxication. They began to neglect their personal hygiene, were confused, had difficulty performing simple tasks and were quarrelsome and occasionally fought. The investigators noted that pathological aspects of some of the subjects' personalities became manifest and some became so depressed that suicide seemed a possibility.

After the subjects had ingested barbiturates on a daily basis for an average of 100 days, these drugs were abruptly withdrawn. Ironically, during the first few hours following drug withdrawal, the signs of chronic intoxication subsided; and the subjects' overall physical and mental states seemed to improve. However, after 12 to 16 hours they began to complain of ill-defined anxieties, abdominal distress and muscular weakness. The most remarkable presentation was the sudden onset of tonic-clonic (grand mal) convulsions between 30 and 115 hours post-drug-withdrawal. Four of five subjects had convulsions; and among these individuals an average of 1 to 3 convulsions were observed. Equally dramatic was the appearance of bizarre psychotic episodes in four of the subjects. These latter manifestations appeared by the third day of withdrawal and had subsided in all cases by the fifteenth day. One individual became so distressed during this period that secobarbital treatment was reinstated and the drug was subsequently withdrawn only slowly.

Overall, the investigators concluded that the manifestions of both chronic barbiturate consumption and subsequent abrupt withdrawal could be life-threatening and were more severe than morphine withdrawal.

b. Meprobamate

Haizlip and Ewing[5] examined the effects of long term meprobamate consumption in two groups of patients which received either 3.2 or 6.4 gm of drug daily while a third group received placebo. When, after 40 days, the drug was replaced with placebo, the attending staff observed objective signs of an abstinence syndrome in forty-four out of forty-seven subjects who received meprobamate throughout the period of chronic dosing. Three patients had convulsions within 36 to 48 hours post-withdrawal, and eight presented manifestations suggestive of delirium tremens.

c. Other Sedative-Hypnotics

By comparison, the consequences of both the long term consumption and subsequent abrupt withdrawal of other sedative-hypnotic agents has been less well investigated. However, the symptoms described in several published case studies are suggestive of those associated with barbiturate intoxication or abstinence. In a review of the subject, Essig[6] noted that the daily consumption of 2.5 to 5 gm of glutethimide produced drowsiness, slurred speech, motor incoordination and impaired memory. Abstinence convulsions also occurred usually appearing between 16 hours and 6 days following glutethimide withdrawal. In one case where 1.5 gm of ethchlorvynol had been consumed daily for months, 3 grand mal convulsions were observed 5 days following drug abstinence. In a second case, 5 convulsions resulted after 2 to 3 gm of ethchlorvynol had been ingested daily for more than 6 months. "Typical" withdrawal signs including convulsions were observed following cessation of the daily consumption of 7.5 to 12 gm of methyprylon.

Three case studies by Swartzburg and his associates[7] demonstrated that the long term daily consumption of 1500 to 2000 milligrams (mg) of methaqualone also led to dependence characterized by the appearance of an abstinence syndrome upon the abrupt withdrawal of this drug. In one of the cases reviewed, the patient experienced at least one grand mal seizure.

KEY STUDIES OF ABUSE POTENTIAL

Despite the detrimental consequences of dependence on the sedative-hypnotics, it seems generally agreed that the development of physical dependence is only a secondary or consequential reinforcer in determining the abuse potential of any addicting compound. Rather, the pleasure-inducing effects produced by the compound appear to be the principal and most common link in dictating abuse liability. The evaluation of this property of the sedative-hypnotics will constitute the focus of the remaining sections of this chapter.

a. Animal Studies

One of the major approaches to evaluating the abuse potential of drugs is to determine whether, with proper training, animals will self-administer the compound of interest. As a further test of the reinforcing properties of the drug, experimental paradigms have been designed to determine whether the animal will *work* in order to receive the drug. To assess these parameters, a progressive-ratio (PR) procedure is typically utilized. With this method the animal is required to repeatedly perform some type of task, e.g., push a lever, in order to receive an injection of drug. Usually, the number of responses required to receive the drug reward are slowly increased as the animal continues to work for the drug. This process continues until the number of responses required to receive the reward exceeds the number that the animal is willing to perform. This number, usually expressed as a ratio of number of responses to reward, thus becomes an objective measure of the desirability of the drug to the animal.

One of the early studies to use PR performance as a measure of the abuse liability of the barbiturates was performed by Griffiths and his coworkers[8] using five male baboons (*Papio anubis*). In this study, the reinforcing properties of secobarbital were compared with those of 2 central stimulants, cocaine and methylphenidate. Once baseline performance was established, the ratio of lever presses required to receive an i.v. drug administration was systematically increased every 7 days. Each time during the day that the drug was administered, a minimum 3 hour time out was instituted before the drug was again available. This process continued with a particular drug until the rate of completing the task to receive drug fell below the criterion (2 or less per day for 3 consecutive days or 4 out of 7 days at a given ratio). The ratio at which the criterion was not met was designated the breaking point. In this study, secobarbital showed a dose-related increase in the breaking point. Further, the two baboons which self-administered the high 12 mg/kg dosage of secobarbital achieved a breaking point equal to that reached when they self-administered 0.8 mg/kg of cocaine.

In a second experiment of very similar design, this research group compared the ability of several barbiturates and benzodiazepines to maintain self-injection behavior that had been initially entrained with cocaine.[9] Chlorpromazine, a phenothiazine tranquilizer with no demonstrable reinforcing ability or abuse potential,[10] was also tested in this study as a control drug. When amobarbital, pentobarbital or secobarbital were provided, the baboons increased their number of injections per day as the dose of the barbiturate was increased up to a mean daily dosage of 5.6 mg/kg. At this dosage level, the average number of daily administrations was comparable to that seen with cocaine. This high and consistent level of barbiturate self-administration was observed in every animal that was tested. By comparison, the benzodiazepines, e.g., clonazepam, clorazepate, diazepam, flurazepam, medazepam or midazolam, resulted in only modest levels of self-administration which were frequently indistinguishable from those observed with placebo. Chlorpromazine was ineffective in maintaining self-administration.

Winger and her associates[11] examined the potency of several barbiturates, e.g., pentobarbital, amobarbital, thiopental, methohexital and barbital, to promote self-administration behavior in 12 rhesus monkeys. Unlike the two above mentioned studies, in this experiment the animals were only allowed to work for drug reward for 3 hours per day but during this time could regulate the amount of barbiturate received by their rate of lever pressing. In this study, each of these drugs was found to maintain lever pressing. As further evidence of the reinforcing power of the barbiturates, if the injected dose was decreased, the monkeys increased their lever pressing in order to receive more administrations of the drug. Overall, an inverse relationship was observed between drug dosage and response rate. Additionally, if, after 7 days of barbiturate-reinforced behavior, saline was abruptly substituted for drug, the monkeys markedly enhanced their rate of responding on the lever. If the drug was not restored within 4 days, the rate of lever pressing fell below that effected by barbiturate reward.

Although it is more difficult to establish than intravenous self-administration, perhaps because of the bitter taste, animals will also orally self-administer barbiturates.[12] After training, three of four baboons consumed larger quantities of methohexital (0.8-6.4 mg/ml) in water than water alone when offered both in a 2 bottle choice condition.[13] Once this behavior was established, it could be replicated if the drug was made available after 1 to 3 months without exposure to methohexital.

Interestingly, in experiments of comparable design and with the use of the same baboons, oral reinforcement could not be established with the benzodiazepines, triazolam or diazepam.[14]

b. Human Studies

1. Barbiturates

Some of the earliest attempts to evaluate the abuse potential of the barbiturates in humans were conducted by Martin and his colleagues.[15,16] In their studies, they compared the effects of single intramuscular injections of morphine and pentobarbital on both physical, e.g., post rotational nystagmus, and psychological parameters. Both subjects and observers were blind to the drugs given. In response to the question "Would you like to take this drug everyday?" subjects responded positively to both morphine and pentobarbital but not to placebo. Dosages of 150, 200 or 250 mg of pentobarbital produced subjective pleasurable effects similar to those of highly euphoric doses of morphine while providing little objective evidence of sedation.

Using similar methodologies, Fraser and Jasinski[17,18] compared the "liking" scores of 3 different barbiturates: pentobarbital (50, 120 or 288 mg/70 kg), secobarbital (75, 180 or 432 mg/70 kg) and phenobarbital (140, 360 or 557.1 mg/70 kg). All 3 drugs produced dose-related increases in both post rotational nystagmus and "liking" scores. Interestingly, both of the pharmacologically short-acting barbiturates, pentobarbital and secobarbital, were about equipotent in affecting these parameters. By comparison, however, phenobarbital was only 1/5 to 1/7 as potent.

Utilizing a markedly different approach, Kliner and Pickens[19] asked one hundred and ninety experienced polydrug users to list the drugs that they had misused and to also indicate the order of preference. In order to participate, the polydrug users must have had experience with at least 3 drugs over a period of at least 2 years. The 11 most frequently listed drugs were ranked. The investigators noted that drug-preference did not seem to be a function of availability or incidence of use and that the rank order seemed to hold over a wide range of dosages and routes of administration. The order of preference was heroin, > amphetamine, > alcohol, > pentobarbital, > secobarbital, > marijuana, > cocaine, > codeine, > diazepam, > LSD, > hashish.

Some of the most thoroughly controlled studies of the abuse potential of the sedative-hypnotics in humans have been performed by Griffiths and his coworkers. Typically, in their studies subjects are required to live in a clinical setting for several weeks during which time dietary intake as well as the consumption of drugs can be carefully controlled. In each of their studies, the subjects are adult male volunteers with histories of sedative drug abuse but who are not drug dependent while participating in the study. In all cases, the subjects and the house staff who dispense the drugs, are kept blind to the identity and the dosage of the drug being administered. Usually, only one or two subjects, involved in the same experiment, are housed in the experimental ward at the same time.

In the earliest of these experiments, subjects were allowed to self-administer up to 10 oral ingestions per day of different dosages of either pentobarbital, diazepam, chlorpromazine or placebo.[20] At the end of each day, the subjects were required to fill out a questionaire indicating whether they felt any effect of the drug and, if so, the relative level of that effect. At the same time, the attending staff filled out a similar questionnaire evaluating the degree of effect of the treatment on the subject. Both pentobarbital and diazepam supported dose-related self-administration. However, the higher, 90 mg/ingestion of pentobarbital maintained levels of self-administration that were substantially and statistically higher than that of the other 2 drugs. Overall, the subjects took 76.1% of the 90mg dosages of pentobarbital that were offered to them as compared to 52.3% of the high dosage (20 mg) of diazepam. These dosages of both drugs were given moderate to high "effect" ratings by both the subjects and the staff. In fact, all 3 drugs at the highest dosage produced observable ataxia and sedation. In contrast to pentobarbital and diazepam, chlorpromazine did not maintain self-administration.

The second study was of a more complex design, consisting of 3 separate experiments.[21] In the first two experiments, the subjects were allowed a single daily choice of 1 of 3 dosages of either pentobarbital (200-900 mg) (experiment 1) or diazepam (50-400 mg) (experiment 2). In the third experiment the subjects had a choice between pentobarbital (400 mg) or diazepam (200 mg). In all 3 of these experiments, there were *no choice* days during which the subjects were required to consume a drug identified by a letter code and *choice* days during which the subjects were presented with the letter codes of 2 drugs, one of which could be selected for ingestion. The subjects were required to fill out several questionnaires assessing drug effect, drug "liking," etc., and the staff filled out an observer-related evaluation of drug effect. In these experiments, pentobarbital produced a clear dose-related increase in both subject- and observer-rated drug effects and in subject-assessed "liking." By comparison, diazepam yielded only modest rating of "liking," and higher dosages were not clearly preferred to lower ones. Further, when given the choice, the subjects consistently selected pentobarbital over diazepam. This preference was evident even though at the dosages ingested both the subjects and the staff rated the depressant effects of these drugs as equivalent. Diazepam did have some reinforcing qualities, however, as it, like pentobarbital, was consistently chosen over placebo.

The subsequent study investigated the ability of pentobarbital to maintain progressive-ratio (PR) performance behavior.[22] As in the animal studies reviewed above, the underlying assumption was that the more reinforcing the drug the more work that the subject would be willing to do in order to receive it. In this experiment either placebo or 1 of 3 dosages of pentobarbital (200, 400 or 600 mg) were available daily. During the first 4 daily sessions, the subject was required to ingest a drug identified as A, B, C or D. They were also told to try to associate the letter identification of the drug with the resulting effect as later they would be given the opportunity to *work* to receive the drug again. After these introductory sessions, on each day the subjects were told the letter name of the drug that was available for that day. However, in order to receive the drug, the subjects were required to complete a work requirement before a specified hour. The work requirement consisted of either riding an exercise bicycle or completing a push button task. If the subject completed the work requirement for a drug, the work requirement was increased at the subsequent session at which that particular drug and dosage was available. In general, the subjects either met the work requirement or did not try at all. The higher dosages of pentobarbital tended to maintain behavior at a higher PR performance than did the lower dosages. Interestingly, there was no descending limb in the dose-reinforcing efficacy function with pentobarbital. This latter observation suggests that the negative manifestions of the highest available dosage of pentobarbital were insufficient to counter the reinforcing qualities of the drug. Further, as in previous studies, pentobarbital produced a dose-related increase in the ratings of both drug effect and drug "liking" provided by both the subjects and the staff.

In an ensuing study Roache and Griffiths compared the ability of pentobarbital and triazolam, a benzodiazepine hypnotic, to impair the performance of simple memory or motor tasks.[23] In this study, pentobarbital was administered in dosages of 100, 200, 400 or 600 mg while triazolam was tested at dosages of 0.5, 1, 2 or 3 mg. Additionally, the subjects and the house staff were both requested to judge the level of impairment produced by the drug treatment. In general, based on the objective measures and on the staff evaluations, the dosage ranges of the two drugs produced roughly equivalent detriments in motor performance. Triazolam appeared to produce a significantly greater impairment of the memory tasks and did so at low non hypnotic doses. Interestingly, when asked to judge their own degree of drug-induced impairment, the subjects reliably estimated the detriment of their performance after treatment with pentobarbital but consistently underestimated the debilitating influence of triazolam. As in earlier studies, when asked to evaluate "liking," "choose again" or "street value," the subjects tended to rate pentobarbital higher than the benzodiazepine.

2. Meprobamate

In 1987, Roache and Griffiths reported the results of their first controlled study of the non-barbiturate, sedative-hypnotic, meprobamate.[24] In this study they compared the effects of this compound with those of lorazepam, a benzodiazepine. In a design similar to other studies, subjects ingested a single daily dose of placebo or drug at 10:00 a.m. Placebo was given for the first 4 to 7 days; then in the ensuing days, 1 of 9 doses of an unidentified test drug or placebo was provided for ingestion. Lorazepam was provided in dosages of 1.5, 3, 6 or 9 mg, and meprobamate was administered in dosages of 600, 1200, 2400 or 3600 mg. In the course of the experiment, all the subjects received all the dosages of both drugs. The staff was asked to estimate the magnitude of the drug effect on the subjects and to take note of the amount of time that the subjects spent sleeping. The subjects were to judge the degree of drug effect, indicate the level of "liking" and evaluate the extent to which the drug made them sleepy or "drunken." Both drugs produced dose-related impairment of task performances which in general were quantitatively similar. Interestingly, however, the subjects were able to estimate more accurately their degree of impairment after meprobamate ingestion than after lorazepam consumption. The two drugs were given similar ratings as to "liking." However, the highest dosage of meprobamate was rated as having a higher street value than any dosage of lorazepam that was tested. Based on the overall results, the investigators concluded that at doses producing similar levels of impairment, meprobamate had an abuse liability at least as great if not greater than that of lorazepam.

3. Methaqualone

Although controlled experiments have not been reported, some case studies suggest anecdotally that methaqualone may possess an abuse potential exceeding that of the barbiturates. One abuser of methaqualone reported it more effective than either secobarbital or amobarbital both as an euphoric and as an hypnotic[25]; another felt it gave a better "high" and more closely approximated the effect of morphine.[7] Out of sixty-six respondents in the Columbus, Ohio area who were known abusers of methaqualone, five commented that "Nothing is quite like a Sopor."[26] Interviews of a number of British heroin addicts, who also abused methaqualone, disclosed that many preferred methaqualone over other hypnotics including barbiturates.[27]

SUMMARY OF ALL STUDIES

The results outlined in the preceding sections of this chapter clearly demonstrate the high abuse potential of the barbiturates. In controlled settings, drug-experienced subjects, blind to the identity of the drug, consistently give the barbiturates high rankings when asked to rate a series of compounds as to "liking," "street value" or "Would you take this drug again?" Further, within a moderate range these drugs appear to become more and more appealing with an increase in administered dosage. Some subjects rate certain dosages of barbiturates as producing a "high" comparable to that produced by euphoric doses of morphine.

The reinforcing properties of these drugs also have been clearly demonstrated in both human and animal studies. Human subjects will work to receive barbiturates and will do more work to receive the drug if the available dosage is increased. In a like manner, nonhuman primates will show similar patterns of lever pressing to receive i.v. injections of the barbiturates.

If only a limited number of injections is allowed per day and a time out period is required between drug administrations, animals show a dose-related increase in the number of times per day that they will complete the criterion required to receive the barbiturate reward. If, on the other hand, the drug is only available for a limited time per day but there are no time outs between opportunities to work for the drug, animals show increased rates of lever pressing if the dosage of the barbiturate is decreased. Further, if the drug is abruptly replaced by vehicle, monkeys initially show a marked increase in lever pressing in an apparent attempt to receive the drug reward.

At least in the human studies, the short-acting barbiturates seem to score higher than the long-acting barbiturates on those subjective criteria that one associates with abuse potential, e.g., drug "liking," etc. This finding is not surprising in the face of general observation of the much wider abuse of secobarbital or pentobarbital as opposed to phenobarbital.[17]

With essentially every subjective criterion believed indicative of abuse liability, the barbiturates score higher than the benzodiazepines. This observation lends credence to the widespread clinical replacement of the barbiturates with benzodiazepine sedative-hypnotics. On the other hand, it is clear from reviewing several of the studies included in this chapter that the benzodiazepines are not free of abuse liability. This may be the case, particularly in the absence of a readily available supply of other more "desirable" drugs. In addition, some of the benzodiazepines appear to enhance subject irritability and seem to impair mental and physical abilities to a greater extent than users are aware.

Unfortunately, other sedative-hypnotics with demonstrated abuse liability have not been evaluated by the same critical methods or compared with barbiturates in the same experimental paradigms. Thus, it is difficult to arrive at an objective determination of the relative abuse potential of these drugs. On the other hand, a review of the literature does provide some hints as to the probable rank order of at least some of the sedative-hypnotics. The Griffiths' group seemed to find it easier to demonstrate a greater abuse potential for the short-acting barbiturates[20,21,23] than for meprobamate[24] when these compounds were individually compared with benzodiazepines. Indirectly, these observations suggest that the short-acting barbiturates have a greater abuse potential than meprobamate. It is more difficult, however, to decide on the relative abuse liabilities of the long-acting barbiturates when compared to meprobamate. A guess made in the absence of hard evidence would be that meprobamate would have greater abuse liability.

The abuse potential of methaqualone also has not been critically evaluated in an experimental setting. However, numerous case studies, clinical reports and results of surveys attest to the considerable abuse liability of this compound. Some subjective information suggests that this drug is more appealing, at least to some abusers, than the barbiturates.

RANK ORDER OF ABUSE POTENTIAL

Within the limitations discussed in the preceding section of this review, this reviewer would rank the sedative-hypnotics in the following order beginning with the most addicting: methaqualone, > short-acting barbiturates, > meprobamate, > sedative-hypnotic benzodiazepines.

BIBLIOGRAPHY

1. Harvey SC. Hypnotics and sedatives. In: Gilman AG, Goodman LS, Rall TW, Murad F, eds. Goodman and Gillman's: The pharmacological basis of therapeutics. New York: Macmillan Publishing Co., 1985: 339-71.

2. Rall TW, Schleifer LS. Drugs effective in the therapy of the epilepsies. In: Gilman AG, Goodman LS, Rall TW, Murad F, eds. Goodman and Gillman's: The pharmacological basis of therapeutics. New York: Macmillan Publishing Co., 1985: 446-72.

3. Bridge TP, Ellinwood EH. Quaalude alley: a one-way street. Am J Psychiatr. 1973; 130: 217-9.

4. Isbell H, Altschul S, Kornetsky CH, Eisenman AJ, Flanary HG, Fraser HF. Chronic barbiturate intoxication. Arch Neurol Psychiatr. 1950; 64: 1-28.

5. Haizlip TM, Ewing JA. Meprobamate habituation: a controlled clinical study. New Engl J Med. 1958; 258: 1181-6.

6. Essig CF. Addiction to nonbarbiturate sedative and tranquilizing drugs. Clin Pharmacol Ther. 1964; 5: 334-43.

7. Swartzburg M, Lieb J, Schwartz AH. Methaqualone withdrawal. Arch Gen Psychiatr. 1973; 29: 46-7.

8. Griffiths RR, Findlew JD, Brady JV, Dolan-Gutcher K, Robinson WW. Comparison of progressive-ratio performance maintained by cocaine, methylphenidate and secobarbital. Psychopharmacologia 1975; 43: 81-3.

9. Griffiths RR, Lukas SE, Bradford LD, Brady JV, Snell JD. Self-injection of barbiturates and benzodiazepines in baboons. Psychopharmacology 1981; 75: 101-9.

10. Deneau G, Yanagita T, Seevers MH. Self-administration of psychoactive substances by the monkey: a measure of psychological dependence. Psychopharmacologia 1969; 16: 30-48.

11. Winger G, Stitzer ML, Woods JH. Barbiturate-reinforce responding in rhesus monkeys: comparison of drugs with different durations of action. J Pharmacol Exp Ther. 1975; 195: 505-14.

12. Ator NA, Griffiths RG. Self-administration of barbiturates and benzodiazepines: a review. Pharmacol Biochem Behav. 1987; 27: 391-8.

13. Ator NA, Griffiths RG. Oral self-administration of methohexital in baboons. Psychopharmacology 1983; 79: 120-5.

14. Griffiths RR, Lamb RJ, Ator NA, Roache JR, Brady JJ. Relative abuse liability of triazolam: experimental assessment in animals and humans. Neurosci Biobehav. Rev. 1985; 9: 133-51.

15. Martin WR, Thompson WO, Fraser HF. Comparison of graded single intramuscular doses of morphine and pentobarbital in man. Clin Pharmacol Ther. 1974; 15: 623-30.

16. McClane TK, Martin WR. Subjective and physiologic effects of morphine, pentobarbital and meprobamate. Clin Pharmacol Ther. 1976; 20: 192-8.

17. Fraser HF, Jasinski DR. The assessment of the abuse potentiality of sedative-hypnotics (depressants). In: Martin WR, ed. Handbook of experimental pharmacology Vol. 45. New York: Springer, 1977: 589-612.

18. Jasinski DR. Clinical evaluation of sedative-hypnotics for abuse potential. In: Thompson T, Unna KR, eds. Predicting dependence liability of stimulant and depressant drugs. Baltimore: University Park Press, 1977: 285-9.

19. Kliner BA, Pickens R. Indicated preference for drugs of abuse. Int J Addict. 1982; 17: 543-7.

20. Griffiths RR, Bigelow G, Liebson I. Human drug self-administration: double blind comparison pentobarbital, diazepam, chlorpromazine and placebo. J Pharmacol Exp Ther. 1979; 210: 301-10.

21. Griffiths RR, Bigelow GE, Liebson I, Kaliszak JE. Drug preference in humans: Double-blind choice comparison of pentobarbital, diazepam and placebo. J Pharmacol Exp Ther. 1980; 215: 649-61.

22. McLoed DR, Griffiths RR. Human progressive-ratio performance: maintenance by pentobarbital. Psychopharmacology 1983; 79: 4-9.

23. Roache JD, Griffiths RR. Comparison of triazolam and pentobarbital: performance impairment, subjective effects and abuse liability. J Pharmacol Exp Ther. 1985; 234: 120-33.

24. Roache JD, Griffiths RR. Lorazepam and meprobamate dose effects in humans: Behavioral effects and abuse liability. J Pharmacol Exp Ther. 1987; 243: 978-88.

25. Slak S. A dozen and two years of methaqualone: a case report. Psycho Rep. 1985; 57: 1097-8.

26. Gerald MC, Schwirian PM. Nonmedical use of methaqualone. Arch Gen Psychiatr. 1973; 28: 627-31.

27. De Alarcon R. Methaqualone. Br Med J. 1969; 1: 122-3.

An Analysis of the Addiction Liability of Nicotine

Allan C. Collins, PhD

SUMMARY. Even though the percent of adults who smoke has been reduced dramatically in the last 20 years, more than 50 million people continue to use tobacco on a daily basis. A majority of these people claim that they would like to stop smoking, but cannot. This review discusses the data suggesting that tobacco smokers are seeking nicotine. The behavioral effects elicited by nicotine and its relative reinforcing properties, as well as the development of tolerance to nicotine and the role of nicotine in the tobacco withdrawal syndrome are discussed. The data indicate that nicotine has addiction liability, but this liability is probably not equal to that of other agents such as cocaine and the opiates.

INTRODUCTION

The health consequences of smoking have received a great deal of attention from the medical community ever since the first Surgeon General's Report on Smoking and Health. The 20th Report of the Surgeon General on the Health Consequences of Smoking (1988) is entitled "Nicotine Addiction."[1] The Report concludes that:

Allan C. Collins is affiliated with the Institute for Behavioral Genetics and Department of Psychology, Campus Box 447, University of Colorado, Boulder, CO 80309.

Dr. Collins is supported in part by a Research Scientist Development Award from the National Institute on Drug Abuse (DA-00116).

83

- Cigarettes and other forms of tobacco are addicting.
- Nicotine is the drug in tobacco that causes addiction.
- The pharmacological and behavioral processes that determine tobacco addiction are similar to those that determine addiction to drugs such as heroin and cocaine.

The Surgeon General's Report is the most comprehensive review of the literature available today; the Report is over 500 pages long, and it reviews thousands of studies. Consequently, the present paper will not attempt to cover the entire literature. The reader is referred to the Surgeon General's Report for this comprehensive review. Rather, this paper will focus on the primary issues related to the potential role of nicotine in regulating tobacco use, and will attempt to discuss some of the areas of dispute generated by the Surgeon General's Report.

EPIDEMIOLOGY OF TOBACCO USE

The use of tobacco products, primarily cigarettes, is widespread in today's society. According to data in the 20th Surgeon General's Report, approximately 26.5% of all Americans 17 years and older were smokers in 1986. This represents 29.5% of all adult males and 23.8% of adult females. While the last 15-20 years have seen dramatic reductions in the per cent of the population using tobacco (51.1% of adult males and 33.3% of females were smokers in 1965), these figures translate into over 50 million people who were smokers in the United States in 1986.

Sex differences in smoking incidence have been reported in virtually every analysis of tobacco use. However, the sex differential is narrowing. During the 1965-1985 time period, a 19.4% reduction was seen in the per cent of males 20 years of age and older who smoked whereas a modest 5.9% reduction was seen in women. In 1965, 51.3% of White males and 59.6% of Black males, 20 years of age and older, were smokers. By 1985, these values had been reduced to 31.8% and 40.6% for White and Black males, respectively. In contrast, 34.5% of White females and 32.7% of Black females were smokers in 1965 whereas 28.3% and 31.6% of these same populations were smokers in 1985. This represents a modest

6.2% decrease in the fraction of White women who smoke and an even more modest 1.1% decrease in Black women.

Apparently, smoking begins relatively early in life. In 1965, 59.2% of all adult males and 41.9% of all adult females, age 20-24 were smokers. Consistent with the trends reported above, these values were reduced in 1985, with 31.0% of males and 32.1% of females in this age group being listed as smokers. Only fragmentary data, using methods that varied from survey to survey, are available for younger age groups, but in the High School Class of 1986, 10.7% of the males and 11.6% of the females reported using a half-pack or more on a daily basis. These trends clearly demonstrate that smoking develops in early adulthood and that the sex differential in tobacco use is disappearing or may even be reversing.

ROLE OF NICOTINE IN TOBACCO USE

While the demographic data provide some indication of the incidence of smoking, these data provide little information about why people smoke or which of the many components of tobacco are being sought. Scientists know surprisingly little about why people smoke, but the evidence is very clear that nicotine is the primary agent that is sought when tobacco is used. Several lines of evidence indicate that nicotine is the most important psychoactive agent in tobacco. For example, cigarette smokers who use low-yield cigarettes smoke more cigarettes per day than do those who smoke high-yield cigarettes, and switching smokers from high-yield to low-yield cigarettes results in an increase in the number of cigarettes smoked.[2] Alternatively, low-yield cigarette smokers increase the rate or depth of puffing, or duration of inhalation or they block filter vents so as to assure delivery of adequate amounts of nicotine.[2,3] These observations have been offered as explanations for the fact that high-yield cigarette smokers maintain blood nicotine levels when the cigarette brand is changed to a low-yield brand. However, nicotine levels are not the only parameters that are reduced in low-yield cigarettes; reduction in tars and other components are also seen. This, and the fact that brand-switching studies have not always resulted in changes in smoking behavior (see Gori and

Lynch[4]) has resulted in some debate as to whether nicotine is the only agent in tobacco that is being sought by smokers.

Perhaps the most convincing argument that nicotine is the sought-after agent in tobacco comes from the observation that pre-treatment with the nicotinic receptor antagonist, mecamylamine, results in an increased consumption of usual brand cigarettes (see Pomerleau et al.,[5] 1987 and the studies cited therein). This increased consumption is accompanied by an increase in plasma nicotine levels and probably represents an attempt by the smoker to overcome the functional blockade of brain nicotinic receptors. In contrast, both oral and intravenous nicotine administration have elicited decreased cigarette smoking in experimental settings where cigarettes were readily available.[6] These data clearly suggest that nicotine is an important factor influencing the amount of tobacco consumed on a daily basis.

Psychoactive Effects of Nicotine

Russell[7] has argued that smoking is a negatively reinforced behavior; i.e., people continue to smoke to avoid withdrawal. This statement begs a very important issue: why do people smoke in the first place? Presumably, nicotine or tobacco is reinforcing, but it is not clear precisely how nicotine elicits its putative reinforcing effects.

Although the data suggest that smokers are seeking nicotine, it is not totally clear as to what behavioral action is being sought. At least theoretically, a psychoactive agent could be reinforcing either because it increases feelings of well being or because it decreases feelings of discomfort, pain or anxiety. Most smokers describe smoking as a pleasurable experience, but it is not totally clear that nicotine has euphoric effects in humans. This is the case because only a very limited number of direct investigations of the behavioral effects of "straight" nicotine have been reported. Johnston[8] injected nicotine intravenously into smokers and nonsmokers; smokers rated the response as pleasurable whereas nonsmokers rated the effects as unpleasant. More recently, Henningfield et al.[6] allowed human volunteers to lever press for the intravenous administration of nicotine. The subjects, most of whom were being treated for some form of substance abuse, rated the nicotine effects as euphoric, as defined by elevations in scores on the Morphine Benzedrine Group scale of the NIDA Addiction Research Center inventory. Those subjects with a drug abuse history also identified the nicotine injections as cocaine. Evidence for dysphoric actions of nicotine were also obtained in this study. These actions became more intense over the course of the experiment and served to limit the number of nicotine injections taken. Thus, it may be that nicotine elicits pleasurable effects at lower doses and unpleasurable effects at higher doses, but it should be noted that the experimental subjects continued to lever press for nicotine even after nausea developed. Most of the subjects did not report a decreased desire to smoke while self administering nicotine, but in the three subjects whose smoking behavior was studied the number of cigarettes smoked and the number of puffs per cigarette were reduced during the self-administration test periods. The studies of Henningfield et al.[6] certainly suggest that intravenous nicotine infusion produces euphoria, but further experiments using additional doses and more subjects, particularly subjects who do not have a history of drug abuse, must be carried out before these findings can be accepted.

Drugs, in general, can also be reinforcing because they decrease pain or anxiety. Nicotine's potential antinociceptive (pain-reducing) effects have been assessed in several experiments. For example, Fertig et al.[9] examined the effects of smoking on pain awareness (subject is aware of pain) and pain endurance (how long subject can endure the pain without responding) using habitual smokers who had been deprived of tobacco for an hour before testing. Pain was induced by placing the subject's forearm in cold (3°) water, and latency between initiation of stimulation and pain perception and removal of the forearm from the water were recorded. Smoking increased the latency for both measures. This study also included an analysis of the effects of nicotine on pain perception and response that used subjects who had been nonsmokers for a minimum of 1 year; nicotine was administered to these subjects in the form of snuff. Once again, latency to pain perception was increased as was pain endurance. These studies clearly argue that, under some circumstances, nicotine may have antinociceptive effects in humans and are consistent with the observation that nicotine has antinociceptive effects in animals.[10]

Nicotine may also decrease anxiety, at least under some circumstances. The use of tobacco products clearly increases when smokers are placed in stressful situations. Significant increases in smoking have been reported in response to a variety of laboratory stressors, including shock, public speaking, aversive white noise, and performing mental arithmetic with competitive pressure (see Pomerleau and Pomerleau[11] for a review). These observations have led to the suggestion that people smoke in an attempt to cope with stress. Although many smokers identify the production of a relaxed state as a motive for smoking, early experiments on the relationship between smoking and anxiety were inconclusive. Problems in demonstrating antianxiety effects of nicotine in smokers may arise because such studies usually use subjects who have been withdrawn from nicotine for several hours which may result in withdrawal-induced increases in anxiety. Pomerleau et al.[12] assessed the effects of a nicotine-containing cigarette and a zero-nicotine cigarette on anxiety produced by presenting the subjects with unsolvable anagrams. The subjects were minimally deprived smokers who refrained from smoking for one hour before testing. The nicotine-containing cigarette elicited a measurable reduction in anxiety as measured by the Spielberger State Anxiety Inventory. Gilbert[13] reviewed the literature in this area a decade ago and concluded that "too few studies have been reported and too many methodological problems are evident in the studies that are available to permit a definite statement about the role of nicotine in altering emotional behavior in humans." This situation has not changed remarkably since Gilbert's review was published.

One of the major problems that hinders progress in this area is most researchers are extremely reticent to give tobacco or nicotine to nonsmokers. Consequently, studies of the behavioral effects of nicotine in humans are frequently confounded by potential withdrawal symptoms. These problems are not encountered in laboratory animal studies. Nicotine injection results in changes in conditioned suppression, emotional freezing and exploratory behaviors that may reflect anxiety-reducing actions in rats.[14] Thus, it may be that nicotine does, indeed, have antianxiety effects in humans, but much additional research using appropriate controls such as non-smokers or ex-smokers may be required to assess fully the potential antianxiety effects of nicotine.

In summary, even though most smokers claim to use tobacco because it gives them pleasure, the studies currently available do not provide unequivocal evidence for nicotine producing reward either via euphoric actions or through reduction of pain, anxiety or negative affect. Even though the study of Henningfield *et al.*[6] indicates that ex-cocaine users recognize nicotine as cocaine, it does not seem probable that a cocaine-like action is dominant in tobacco smokers, perhaps because smokers do not attain the necessary brain levels of nicotine to elicit cocaine-like actions. Similarly, questions regarding potential analgesic or antianxiety effects of nicotine persist. Consequently, the reasons why smokers find tobacco or nicotine pleasurable remain unclear.

FACTORS THAT INFLUENCE SMOKING

Environmental Factors

Tobacco products are readily available, yet not every person chooses to smoke or chew tobacco. This, of course, indicates that individuals differ either in the environmental or genetic factors that regulate smoking. As noted above, smokers generally increase their use of tobacco products when placed in stressful environments. Similarly, it is very clear that an association exists between alcoholic beverage consumption and cigarette smoking. A greater fraction of the alcoholic population smoke than do nonalcoholics and cigarette smokers who have been diagnosed as alcoholics smoke more cigarettes per day than do nonalcoholic cigarette smokers (see Henningfield et al.[15] and Mello et al.,[16] for a review of this literature). Laboratory studies utilizing alcoholic and nonalcoholic subjects indicate that as alcohol consumption increases, so does to-bacco use.[15,16]

Genetic Factors

In chapter 5 of the 20th Surgeon General's Report, considerable attention is given to the fact that individuals differ in smoking behavior. This pattern is highly reminiscent of the pattern seen with alcohol. A host of studies have indicated that alcoholism is familial and adoption studies have demonstrated that the drinking behavior of the adoptee more closely resembles the drinking behavior of the biological parent. Although not nearly as well studied, several reports indicate that a genetic predisposition may contribute to tobacco use. Fisher[17,18] studied the smoking behavior of identical twins and noted that concordance for smoking behavior (whether both twins were smokers or nonsmokers) was greater in a population of monozygotic (identical) twins than was the concordance in dizygotic twins. Fisher argued that the greater concordance for smoking behavior seen in the identical twin pairs indicates that tobacco use is influenced by genetic factors. Subsequent studies of smoking behavior in monozygotic and dizygotic twins have supported Fisher's arguments (see Gurling et al.,[19] for original contributions as well as a review of this literature). As is the case with alcohol use and abuse, the human genetic studies do not point towards a potential cause of smoking; the data indicate only that some genetic factor(s) either promote or inhibit tobacco use.

REINFORCING PROPERTIES OF NICOTINE: FINDINGS FROM BASIC RESEARCH

Primarily because of ethical considerations, very few investigators have attempted to assess the potential rewarding or reinforcing properties of nicotine in humans. Assessing the potential reinforcing effects of drugs, in general, has been developed to a high degree in laboratory animals. Three approaches have been used: the drug self-administration procedures which generally involve rewarding an animal for pressing the appropriate lever, conditioned place preference and drug discrimination. All of these strategies have been used to assess the potential reinforcing properties of nicotine, and equivocal results have been obtained.

Self-Administration Studies

Self-administration studies have classically been used to assess whether an agent has reinforcing properties. Most of these studies are done in animals, but occasionally humans are used. As mentioned above, Henningfield et al.[6] have successfully demonstrated that human volunteers, most of whom were being treated for substance abuse, will press a lever to attain an intravenous nicotine reward. These subjects described the effects elicited as pleasurable, and those with a substance abuse history likened the response to that elicited by cocaine.

Studies of nicotine self-administration by animals show that nicotine may act as a reinforcer, but its efficacy and the range of conditions under which it will be self-administered are limited. Nicotine will be self-administered by rats, squirrel monkeys, rhesus monkeys, baboons and dogs (see Henningfield[3] and Clarke[20] for recent reviews). Nicotine self-administration is reduced or eliminated by treatment with high doses of the nicotinic antagonist mecamylamine.[21]

While these studies have all demonstrated that animals will self-administer nicotine, the evidence suggests that self-administration is not readily attained. In general, long periods of training are required and response rates are quite low. In addition, factors other than drug or drug dose influence the response rate. For example, Lang et al.[22] have shown that rats can be trained to self-administer nicotine only if they are maintained at a reduced body weight. Similarly, rats that are exposed to stress will self-inject nicotine more readily than will nonstressed rats.[23]

Goldberg's[21] studies of nicotine self-administration by squirrel monkeys are probably the most effective demonstrations that animals will self-administer nicotine. These studies were published shortly after Griffiths et al.[24] had concluded that nicotine is a weak reinforcer when compared to other drugs of abuse. Goldberg and co-workers used second-order schedules of reinforcement (every tenth response resulted in the presentation of a brief visual stimulus which was occasionally paired with an injection of 0.03 mg/kg nicotine). Most other investigators have used simple or continuous schedules of reinforcement. Using the second-order schedule prevented injections from occurring at interinjection intervals of 5 min or less. Too frequent injections, or too high a dose, results in nicotine being aversive.

Squirrel monkeys will also consume nicotine in high doses when it is given orally.[25] However, this occurs only if noncontingent tail shocks are administered. In control sessions, subjects drink most of their fluid from water-only bottles.

Risner and Goldberg[26] were also successful in detecting significant self-administration of nicotine in beagle dogs using a procedure that involved a fixed ratio of 15 (15 lever presses for each drug injection) and a 4 minute time out period immediately after injection. This study showed: peak rates of responding were about 0.3 responses/sec (higher rates were maintained by cocaine); response rates increased with dose and then decreased at higher nicotine doses; and response rates for nicotine, but not cocaine, were reduced by pretreatment with mecamylamine.

All of these studies indicate that, under appropriate circumstances, nicotine can serve as a reinforcer. However, the dose must be controlled and time between doses may be critical. In addition, the environment may also play a critical role in determining whether nicotine has reinforcing properties or not. The effects of environmental variables such as feeding status and stress on self-administration led Balfour[27] to argue that nicotine does not act as a particularly effective positive reward in a "neutral" environment but can act as a positive reinforcer in situations in which it alleviates some unpleasant physiological response. Similarly, Henningfield[3] suggested "that nicotine serves as a reinforcer under a more limited range of conditions than do other reinforcers and that its strength is more related to environmental stimuli than is the case for other drugs of abuse." This reviewer is unaware of any published reports that have appeared recently that would alter the situation. Thus, nicotine can serve as a reinforcer in laboratory animals, as measured by self-administration studies, but the range of conditions over which this reinforcing effect may be observed is less than that seen for agents such as opiates and cocaine.

Conditioned Place Preference Studies

Conditioned place preference is a new procedure that has been used to evaluate the rewarding properties of psychoactive agents. At least conceptually, it is a simpler procedure than is the self-administration paradigm. Conditioned place preference is achieved by repeatedly injecting the subjects with the test drug and placing them in one chamber of a two or three chamber test apparatus and injecting them with saline and placing them in another chamber of the test apparatus. Thus, the animal is trained to associate one chamber with the drug and another with saline. On the test day the animal is simply placed in the test apparatus and the barrier separating the two training chambers is removed. The fraction of the test time spent in the drug- and saline-trained chambers is measured. Fudala et al.[28] were successful in demonstrating conditioned place preference for nicotine in the rat, but Clarke and Fibiger[29] were not. We (unpublished) have not been successful in developing nicotine-induced conditioned place preference in any of three inbred mouse strains. Consequently, it does not seem as though this method of measuring drug reinforcement is likely to yield reliably positive results for nicotine.

Drug Discrimination Studies

Another method that has proven useful in assessing pharmacological actions of drugs in animals is the drug discrimination paradigm. Animals are taught to make one operant response following injection with the prototype drug and another response following saline. Most often this involves pressing one lever following drug and another following saline. Rats can be trained to discriminate nicotine (see Stolerman et al.,[30] for a review). This behavior can be blocked by mecamylamine and hexamethonium, if the latter drug is injected centrally.[30] All of the studies to date indicate that rats recognize only other nicotinic agonists as nicotine with the possible exception of d-amphetamine. Other agents such as opiates, cocaine, barbiturates etc. were not recognized as nicotine-like in any of these studies which suggests that nicotine's actions are not similar to those elicited by these other agents.

TOLERANCE TO NICOTINE

The continual use of many drugs is often accompanied by tolerance, i.e., a reduced intensity of response following the administration of a given dose of the drug. The development of tolerance, particularly to toxic or dysphoric effects of a drug, may be critical to achieving drug dependence in that such tolerance could facilitate increasing dose and dose frequency. Tolerance to the actions of nicotine has been well established both in humans and animals. In some cases, tolerance develops within a dose or two (tachyphylaxis), in other cases more prolonged exposure to nicotine is required (chronic tolerance).

Tachyphylaxis

Only a limited number of studies have attempted to determine whether tachyphylaxis to nicotine's actions occurs in humans even though anecdotal evidence indicates that it must. Smokers frequently report that the first cigarette of the day is more pleasurable and that subsequent cigarettes are "tasteless."[3] Rosenberg et al.[31] measured the effects of intravenous nicotine administration on heart rate, blood pressure and arousal level by injecting six healthy smokers with six series of nicotine injections, spaced 30 minutes apart. A pleasant sensation was reported by the subjects after the first injections, but not thereafter. Similarly, nicotine elicited increases in blood pressure and heart rate after the first injections, but not thereafter. More recently, Henningfield[3] also reported rapid loss of "liking" responses to i.v. nicotine during chronic injections as well as reduced sensitivity to the effects of nicotine on heart rate and blood pressure.[32] The amount of tolerance lost between cycles is influenced by the time period between nicotine administrations and tolerance is very quickly re-established.

A sizable literature indicates that tolerance to the effects of nicotine develops in animals with as little as one dose. Pretreatment with a single dose of nicotine results in reduced sensitivity to: the lethal effects of nicotine in the mouse, the locomotor depressant activity of nicotine in the rat and mouse, the hypothermic effects of nicotine in the cat, altered discharge of lateral geniculate neurons in the cat, and blood pressure elevation in rats.[20] In addition, tachyphylaxis to nicotine-induced seizures occurs in the mouse.[33] Tachyphylaxis to nicotine's seizure-inducing effects develops within 15 minutes after pretreatment with nicotine and it disappears within 60 minutes. Furthermore, tachyphylaxis to this effect of nicotine is seen in some mouse strains, but not in others.

Although tachyphylaxis to the effects of nicotine has been demonstrated for many of nicotine's effects, potential explanations for this phenomenon have not been forthcoming. Barrass et al.[34] have suggested that a nicotine metabolite may block nicotine receptors in the CNS, and we[33] have suggested that nicotinic receptor desensitization may underlie tachyphylaxis to nicotine's actions, but these suggestions must be labeled as speculative because there is no direct evidence that nicotine metabolites bind with high affinity to brain nicotinic receptors or that these receptors desensitize.

Chronic Tolerance

Retrospective reports by smokers indicate that the first few cigarettes induced feelings of nausea, dizziness, vomiting, headache, and dysphoria.[7] These symptoms disappear with continued smoking, but tolerance is not complete since symptoms of nicotine toxicity reappear when smokers increase their tobacco consumption by as little as 50%.[35]

The development of chronic tolerance to nicotine has been established using several different behavioral and physiological tests as measures of drug effect. For example, tolerance to the locomotor activity depressing effects of nicotine has been clearly established in rats following chronic injections and mice display a reduced locomotor depression following chronic nicotine injections or chronic intravenous infusions.[36,37,38] Tolerance also develops to nicotine's effects on respiratory rate, heart rate, and body temperature in the mouse. This tolerance increases with nicotine dose[36] and varies among inbred mouse strains.[36,38] Tolerance to nicotine in the mouse is paralleled by an increase in the number of brain nicotinic receptors. Similarly, a greater number of nicotinic receptors has recently been reported for brain tissue obtained from human smokers.[39] We[36] have suggested that a high fraction of these up-regulated nicotinic receptors are inactivated or desensitized based on a combination of behavioral and biochemical evidence.

WITHDRAWAL FROM NICOTINE

Human Studies

The literature relating to withdrawal from tobacco is extraordinarily large. No attempt will be made to summarize this literature here. Rather, the role of nicotine in tobacco withdrawal will be emphasized.

The tobacco withdrawal syndrome, as described in the Diagnostic and Statistical Manual (DSM III-R, APA 1987), is complex. Included among the dominant symptoms are: (1) craving for nicotine, (2) irritability, frustration or anger, (3) anxiety, (4) difficulty concentrating, (5) restlessness, (6) decreased heart rate, and (7) increased appetite or weight gain. These symptoms vary in intensity during the course of withdrawal and withdrawal symptoms may be seen as long as 14 days after smoking has been terminated.[40]

The data concerning the possible role of nicotine in tobacco withdrawal are complicated. For example, some studies have indicated that smokers who undergo abrupt cessation experience less severe withdrawal than do smokers who only partially reduce their daily use of tobacco.[41] Other studies indicate that abrupt, total cessation results in a more severe withdrawal syndrome.[42] Subjects in this latter study who reduced the number of cigarettes smoked by 50% or switched to low-yield cigarettes failed to exhibit a detectable withdrawal syndrome.

Most of the studies of tobacco withdrawal have not measured blood nicotine levels, but Hatsukami et al.[43] did measure nicotine levels before and after stopping tobacco use. Subjects' reports of craving for cigarettes were related to nicotine levels. No significant relationship between nicotine levels and changes in heart rate, caloric intake, and reports of confusion and number of awakenings during sleep were detected following smoking cessation. On the other hand, nicotine administration, in gum, reduced irritability, anxiety, difficulty in concentrating, restlessness, impatience, and somatic complaints in subjects undergoing withdrawal.[44] Nicotine did not reduce the increases in cigarette craving, hunger, eating, insomnia, tremulousness or supine heart rate after cessation. Several other studies (see, for example, West et al.,[45]) have also reported that nicotine gum attenuates some, but not all, tobacco withdrawal symptoms. In particular, nicotine gum has not replicably reduced the desire to smoke.

These findings are puzzling if the nicotine addiction theory is correct. If human tobacco smokers are addicted to nicotine, partial reductions in blood nicotine levels should reproducibly result in the appearance of a withdrawal syndrome; this syndrome should be more severe in totally abstinent individuals. Conversely, nicotine replacement should eliminate or minimize the most significant withdrawal symptoms, especially craving. As noted above, recent findings do not uniformly reach these expectations; the data are not consistent from study to study.

One potential explanation for the confusion that exists in this literature is that individual differences in withdrawal have been commented on, but largely ignored. Virtually every study reports sizable standard errors, and two studies[46,47] comment specifically on the large individual differences in withdrawal severity. Nonetheless, the assumption is made that an habitual smoker is automatically addicted to tobacco. This may be as fallacious as is the assumption that everyone who drinks alcohol on a daily basis is addicted to alcohol. It may be that some tobacco smokers can use nicotine chronically without becoming fully dependent on it.

Animal Studies

Very few investigators have attempted to systematically measure a nicotine withdrawal syndrome in laboratory animals. The only positive results reported to date are from the studies of Gruneberg et al.[48,49] who have demonstrated that rats undergoing withdrawal from chronic nicotine administration increase their intake of sweet food and gain weight; no such effect is seen if low calorie, bland foods are the only food sources available.[48] Additional studies are clearly needed in this area, particularly if quantitative assessments of withdrawal are to be made.

CONCLUSIONS

Because there are currently more than 50 million people in the United States who are daily users of tobacco and because many of these individuals claim they would like to quit, but cannot, it seems reasonable to place nicotine on the list of substances with addiction liability; to do anything other than this would be foolish. The 20th Report of the Surgeon General concluded that the addiction liability of nicotine is equal to that of cocaine or heroin. In the view of this reviewer, the literature does not support this classification. Nicotine does not have profound euphoric effects, at least at the doses that are normally used. Smokers can function in society very well and may actually exhibit an increase in alertness and ability to concentrate. Animals will self-administer nicotine, but the circumstances under which self-administration will occur are clearly more limited than are those that influence cocaine and opiate self-administration. Thus, if drug self-administration by animals is an adequate model for human drug-seeking behavior, it seems probable that nicotine is rewarding only under relatively well specified circumstances.

Tolerance develops to many of the actions of nicotine. In smokers and in laboratory animals this tolerance appears to be relatively small compared to other drugs; two-fold differences in the doses required to elicit measurable effects are seen between smokers and nonsmokers. While tolerance, in and of itself, is probably not a cause of dependence, it is likely that the greater the tolerance, particularly to toxic actions, the larger the dose that can be consumed.

The observation that some smokers, but not all smokers, exhibit a withdrawal syndrome when smoking is discontinued may be important from a practical viewpoint. Evaluating drug dependence is probably done most readily in subjects who are genuinely dependent on the drug. In addition, the observation that nicotine gum does not uniformly reverse all of the withdrawal symptoms, particularly craving, suggests that more than nicotine is involved in tobacco dependence unless the pharmacokinetics of nicotine administration are vastly different when smoking and gum chewing are compared. These differences may account for the partial success that nicotine-containing gum seems to have in reducing tobacco withdrawal symptoms.

In summary, nicotine is clearly not without addiction potential; far too many people continue to use tobacco even though they claim that they would like to stop. However, nicotine's relative abuse potential is probably not equivalent to that of cocaine and heroin. If it was, the data would be more consistent in the self-administration and withdrawal areas.

REFERENCES

1. Report of the Surgeon General of the United States. *The Health Consequences of Smoking: Nicotine Addiction.* US Department of Health and Human Services, Office of Smoking and Health, Rockville, MD 20857.

2. Zacny JP, Stitzer ML. Cigarette brand-switching: Effects on smoke exposure and smoking behavior. J Pharmacol Exp Ther. 1988; 246:619-627.

3. Henningfield JE. Behavioral pharmacology of cigarette smoking. Adv Behav Pharmacol. 1984; 4:131-210.

4. Gori GB, Lynch CJ. Analytical cigarette yields as predictors of smoke bioavailability. Regul Toxicol Pharmacol. 1985; 5:314-326.

5. Pomerleau CS, Pomerleau OF, Majchrzak MJ. Mecamylamine pretreatment increases subsequent nicotine self-administration as indicated by changes in plasma nicotine level. Psychopharmacology 1987; 91:391-3.

6. Henningfield JE, Miyasoto K, Jasinski DR. Cigarette smokers self-administer intravenous nicotine. Pharmacol Biochem Behav. 1983; 19:887-890.

7. Russell MAH. Smoking problems: An overview. In: Jarvik M, Cullin J, Gritz E, Vogt T, West L (eds) *Research on Smoking Behavior.* NIDA Research Monograph 17. National Institute on Drug Abuse. 1977:13-34.

8. Johnston LM. Tobacco smoking and nicotine. Lancet 1942; 2:742.

9. Fertig JB, Pomerleau OF, Sanders B. Nicotine-produced antinociception in minimally deprived smokers and ex-smokers. Addict Behav 1986; 11:239-248.

10. Tripathi H, Martin B, Aceto M. Nicotine-induced antinociception in rats and mice: Correlations with nicotine brain levels. J Pharmacol Exp Ther. 1982; 221:91-6.

11. Pomerleau CS, Pomerleau OF. The effects of a psychological stressor on cigarette smoking and subsequent behavioral and physiological responses. Psychophysiology 1987; 24:278-285.

12. Pomerleau OF, Turk DC, Fertig JB. The effects of cigarette smoking on pain and anxiety. Addict Behav. 1984; 9:265-271.

13. Gilbert DG. Paradoxical tranquilizing and emotion-reducing effects of nicotine. Psychol Bull. 1979; 86:643-661.

14. Fleming JC, Broadhurst PL. The effects of nicotine on two-way avoidance

conditioning in bidirectionally selected strains of rats. Psychopharmacologia 1975; 42:147-152.

15. Henningfield JE, Chait LD, Griffiths RR. Effects of ethanol on cigarette smoking by volunteers without histories of alcoholism. Psychopharmacology 1984; 82:1-5.

16. Mello NK, Mendelsohn JH, Palmieri SL. Cigarette smoking by women: Interactions with alcohol use. Psychopharmacology 1987; 93:8-15.

17. Fisher RA. Lung cancer and cigarettes? Nature 1958a; 182:108.

18. Fisher RA. Cancer and smoking. Nature 1958b; 182:596.

19. Gurling HMD, Grant S, Dangl J. The genetic and cultural transmission of alcohol use, alcoholism, cigarette smoking and coffee drinking: A review and an example using a log linear cultural transmission model. Brit J Addict 1985; 80:269-279.

20. Clarke PBS. Nicotine and smoking: A perspective from animal studies. Psychopharmacology 1987; 92:135-143.

21. Goldberg SR, Spealman RA, Goldberg DM. Persistent high rate behavior maintained by intravenous self-administration of nicotine. Science 1981; 214:573-5.

22. Lang WJ, Jatiff AA, McQueen A, Singer G. Self-administration of nicotine with and without a food delivery schedule. Pharmacol Biochem Behav. 1977; 7:65-70.

23. Hanson HM, Ivester CA, Morton BR. Nicotine self-administration in rats. In: Krasnegor NA (ed) *Cigarette Smoking as a Dependence Process*. NIDA Research Monograph 23. National Institute on Drug Abuse. 1979:70-90.

24. Griffiths RR, Brady JV, Bradford LD. Predicting the abuse liability of drugs with animal drug self-administration procedures: Psychomotor stimulants and hallucinogens. In: Thompson T, Dews PB (eds) *Advances in Behavioral Pharmacology* (Vol2) New York, Academic Press 1979:163-208.

25. Hutchinson RR, Emley GS. Aversive stimulation produces nicotine ingestion in squirrel monkeys. Psychol Rec. 1985; 35:491-502.

26. Risner ME, Goldberg SR. A comparison of nicotine and cocaine self-administration in the dog: Fixed-ratio and progressive-ratio schedules of intravenous drug infusion. J Pharmacol Exp Ther. 1983; 224:319-326.

27. Balfour DJK. The pharmacology of nicotine dependence: A working hypothesis. Pharmac Ther. 1982; 15:239-250.

28. Fudala PJ, Teoh KW, Iwamoto ET. Pharmacological characterization of nicotine-induced conditioned place preference. Pharmacol Biochem Behav. 1985; 22:237-241.

29. Clarke PBS, Fibiger HC. Apparent absence of nicotine-induced conditioned place preference in rats. Psychopharmacology 1987; 92:84-88.

30. Stolerman IP, Garcha HS, Pratt JA, Kumar R. Role of training dose in discrimination of nicotine and related compounds by rats. Psychopharmacology 1984; 84:413-19.

31. Rosenberg J, Benowitz NL, Jacob B, Wilson KM. Disposition kinetics and effects of intravenous nicotine. Clin Pharmacol Ther. 1980; 28:517-522.

32. Benowitz NL, Jacob P, Jones RT, Rosenberg J. Interindividual variability in the metabolism and cardiovascular effects of nicotine in man. J Pharmacol Exp Ther 1982; 221:368-372.

33. Miner LL, Collins AC. Effect of nicotine pretreatment on nicotine-induced seizures. Pharmacol Biochem Behav. 1988; 29:375-380.

34. Barrass BC, Blackburn JW, Brimblecomb RW, Rich P. Modification of nicotine toxicity by pretreatment with different drugs. Biochem Pharmacol. 1969; 18:2145-2152.

35. Danaher, BG. Research on rapid smoking: Interim summary and recommendations. Addict Behav 1977; 2:151-166.

36. Marks MJ, Burch JB, Collins AC. Effects of chronic nicotine infusion on tolerance development and cholinergic receptors. J Pharmacol Exp Ther. 1983; 226:806-816.

37. Marks MJ, Stitzel JA, Collins AC. A dose-response analysis of nicotine tolerance and receptor changes in two inbred mouse strains. J Pharmacol Exp Ther. 1986; 239:358-364.

38. Marks MJ, Stitzel JA, Collins AC. Influence of kinetics of nicotine administration on tolerance development and receptor levels. Pharmacol Biochem Behav. 1987; 27:505-512.

39. Benwell MEM, Balfour DJK, Anderson JM. Evidence that tobacco smoking increases the density of (-)-[³H]nicotine binding sites in human brain. J Neurochem 1988; 50:1243-7.

40. Shiffman SM, Jarvik ME. Smoking withdrawal symptoms in two weeks of abstinence. Psychopharmacology 1976; 50:35-9.

41. Manley R, Boland F. Side-effects and weight gain following a smoking cessation program. Addict Behav. 1983; 8:375-380.

42. Hatsukami DK, Dahlgren L, Zimmerman R, Hughes JR. Symptoms of tobacco withdrawal from total cigarette cessation versus partial cigarette reduction. Psychopharmacology 1988; 94:242-7.

43. Hatsukami DK, Hughes JR, Pickens RW. Blood nicotine, smoke exposure and tobacco withdrawal symptoms. Addict Behav, 1985; 10:413-417.

44. Hughes JR, Hatsukami DK, Pickens RW, Krahn D, Malin S, Luknic A. Effect of nicotine on the tobacco withdrawal syndrome. Psychopharmacology 1984; 83:82-7.

45. Hatsukami DK, Hughes JR, Pickens RW, Svikis D. Tobacco withdrawal symptoms: An experimental analysis. Psychopharmacology 1984; 84:231-6.

46. West RJ, Hajek P, Belcher M. Which smokers report most relief from craving when using nicotine gum? Psychopharmacology 1986; 89:189-191.

47. West R, Russell MAH. Loss of acute nicotine tolerance and severity of cigarette withdrawal. Psychopharmacology 1988; 94:563-5.

48. Gruneberg NE, Bowen DJ, Morse DE. Effects of nicotine on body weight and food consumption in rats. Psychopharmacology 1984; 83:93-8.

49. Gruneberg NE, Bowen DJ, Maycock DA, Nespor SM. The importance of sweet taste and caloric contents in the effects of nicotine on specific food consumption. Psychopharmacology 1985; 87:198-203.

Addiction Potential of Benzodiazepines and Non-Benzodiazepine Anxiolytics

John D. Roache, PhD

SUMMARY. This paper reviews the addiction potential of all benzodiazepines currently available in the U.S.A. as well as several non-benzodiazepine anxiolytic drugs. Addiction potential was assessed by separately considering the potential for these drugs to produce three different phenomena of addiction; namely, physical dependence, psychological dependence and deleterious consequences. This review focuses on human studies conducted with research volunteers outside the therapeutic context and also on clinical studies conducted with patients receiving treatment in the therapeutic context. It is concluded that benzodiazepines have a reduced addiction potential in comparison to the predecessor barbiturates. Conclusions regarding the relative addiction potential of several non-benzodiazepine anxiolytics are difficult due to a paucity of data; however limited evidence suggests a reduced addiction potential for several of these compounds. Within the benzodiazepine class, qualitative differences in addiction potential between individual drugs are not well established.

INTRODUCTION

In reviewing the addiction potential of benzodiazepines (BZ's) and non-BZ anxiolytics, one must retain as a caveat that recurring cycles have appeared throughout the historical development of different CNS depressants.[1] Since the early use of bromide salts in the

John D. Roache is affiliated with the Department of Psychiatry and Behavioral Sciences and Department of Pharmacology, University of Texas Medical School at Houston, and the Substance Abuse Research Group, University of Texas Mental Sciences Institute. Correspondence may be addressed to the author at the University of Texas Mental Sciences Institute, Substance Abuse Research, Room 342, 1300 Moursund Avenue, Houston, TX 77030.

103

nineteenth century, the introduction of each successive generation of psychosedative has been heralded as a major innovation resulting in improved efficacy with reduced side effects. Each of the drugs successively developed, including paraldehyde, chloral hydrate, barbiturates, meprobamate and the BZ's, probably represent improvements in efficacy and/or safety; however, the potential for abuse and addiction has been recognized belatedly in each case. The barbiturates fell into disfavor in the late 1950's as their potential for abuse and physical dependence was recognized. The BZ's have now replaced the barbiturates for the treatment of anxiety disorders. Compared to the barbiturates, BZ's are considered safer and more effective with fewer side effects. However, BZ's were once thought to not cause addiction. Now, more than 25 years following the introduction of chlordiazepoxide, we have finally begun to recognize the addiction potential of the BZ's.

DEFINITIONS OF ADDICTION POTENTIAL

Although the term addiction has long been considered by the lay public to refer to an intense devotion to a bad habit or a regular over-reliance upon a drug, the medical and scientific communities have had a much less clear view of the meaning of addiction. Early clinical researchers attempted to operationalize the term to describe the state of chronic intoxication to opioids or barbiturates which was associated with mostly physiological signs observed upon cessation of drug treatment. With this definition, drugs which did not produce fairly profound physiological withdrawal signs (e.g., cocaine) were unfortunately considered by some as non-addicting. In order to standardize definitions and allow for compulsive drug taking which occurs in the absence of strong physiological withdrawal signs, the World Health Organization abandoned the term addiction in favor of the term "drug dependence" which was defined as: "A state, psychic and sometimes also physical, which results from the interaction between a living organism and a drug, which is characterized by behavioral and other responses that always include compulsion to take the drug on a continuous or periodic basis in order to experience its psychic effects and sometimes to avoid the discomfort of its absence. Tolerance may be present." This definition of drug dependence commonly is subdivided into the categories of "physical dependence" to describe the state evidenced by withdrawal symptoms observed in the chronic user upon drug abstinence and "psychological dependence" to refer to the psychic drive or emotional state evidenced by the intense reliance upon and compulsive use of the substance. Whereas scientists can operationally define drug dependence, drug abuse and drug addiction are socially defined terms which refer to socially unacceptable forms of drug use or drug dependence, respectively. While variables influencing social attitudes are not always clear, Western society generally would define drug dependence as addiction when regular drug self-ingestion occurs in a pattern which is detrimental or interferes with social function.[2] The medical community and the lay public need information on each of the components involved in the definition of an addictive substance in order to make informed decisions and judgments regarding the use and control of these substances. Therefore, this paper will provide information on the *addiction potential* of BZ's and other anxiolytics by separately assessing their potential for *physical dependence, psychological dependence* and *deleterious consequences or socially detrimental effects*. It should be noted that the Diagnostic and Statistical Manual (DSM III-R) of the American Psychiatric Association incorporates the concept of social impairment within the definition of substance dependence. However, it may be worthwhile to maintain a distinction between the terms addiction and dependence because physical dependence could develop without producing socially injurious effects and psychological dependence may occur in such a way that society would not consider it harmful (e.g., regular caffeine use).[2] Finally, consistent with the distinctions made in DSM III-R, substance *abuse* is distinguished from dependence (or addiction) in that abuse refers to a harmful pattern of drug self-ingestion which is not so extreme as to be considered drug dependence.

ANXIOLYTICS TO BE DISCUSSED

As the term "anxiolytic" suggests, this paper should address those agents which are effective in the treatment of anxiety disorders. Historically, a variety of CNS depressants including bromide salts, paraldehyde, choral hydrate, meprobamate and barbiturates have been used to sedate or tranquilize the emotionally aroused patient. With the ubiquitous use of BZ's in the last 25 years, these drugs have largely replaced other types of pharmacotherapy and have become almost synonymous with the term anxiolytic. This term has been used to distinguish the presumably anxio-selective actions of BZ minor tranquilizers from the major tranquilizer phenothiazine or buterophenone neuroleptics. Other than the BZ's, several types of drugs have been used to treat anxiety including neuroleptics, antidepressants, antihistamines and adrenergic blockers; however, with few exceptions, BZ anxiolytics are considered superior in efficacy.[3] Several recent developments in pharmacopsychiatry have begun to shake the previously unchallenged position of BZ's in the treatment of anxiety disorders. In one development, Panic Disorder was redefined as a distinct diagnostic disorder which is responsive to tricyclic and monoamine oxidase inhibitor antidepressants. This, coupled with the recent use of imipramine in anxiety disorders and BZ's in affective and panic disorders,[3] has muddled the distinctions between the drug classes used to treat anxiety and depression. Finally, the introduction of buspirone as a novel anxiolytic has challenged theories regarding the biological basis of anxiety and presumably has ushered in a new generation of anxiolytic agents which are structurally unrelated to the BZ's and do not act through BZ receptors.[3,4]

Since their introduction in the early 1960's, BZ's increasingly have replaced the barbiturates for various psychotherapeutic purposes; barbiturates are no longer used for anxiolytic indications. Perhaps it is not surprising that the majority of BZ prescriptions are written by non-psychiatric physicians for the symptomatic treatment of a variety of illnesses manifesting anxiety and insomnia.[5] BZ's have been among the most widely prescribed drugs in the world and diazepam has been the most frequently prescribed BZ. Worldwide, BZ use reached a peak in the mid 1970's when concerns regarding an over-medicated society caused a re-evaluation of prescribing practices[5,6]; prescription rates for BZ's and other sedatives generally have been declining ever since. During the same period, there was an increasing recognition of BZ addiction occurring within the therapeutic context. Due to concerns regarding BZ overuse and addiction, there is now an interest in the use of non-BZ compounds and also in the development of new anxiolytics with reduced addiction potential.

In this paper, the addiction potential of BZ's and other non-BZ anxiolytics will be assessed mostly through an examination of studies conducted in human research volunteers and patients receiving treatment in the therapeutic context. Most of these data will refer to BZ's in general and diazepam in particular since these have been the most widely used and studied drugs. However, due to an interest in the use of non-BZ's or some of the newer BZ anxiolytics, data regarding each of the individual drugs listed in Table 1 will be introduced where possible. The thirteen BZ's currently approved for use in the U.S. are categorized according to their pharmacokinetic elimination profiles: six BZ's produce active N-desalkyl metabolites which are slowly-eliminated, three of which (chlordiazepoxide, diazepam and flurazepam) are active parent compounds and three (clorazepate, halazepam and prazepam) are inactive pro-drugs which are converted to the active metabolites; five BZ's (alprazolam, clonazepam, lorazepam, oxazepam, and temazepam) have intermediate elimination profiles; and two BZ's (midazolam and triazolam) have very rapid elimination profiles. The non-BZ compounds which are available for use as anxiolytics[3] are also listed in Table 1. Of these, the beta-blockers (e.g., propranolol) have not proved useful although there has been a renewed interest in the use of antidepressants (e.g., doxepin and imipramine). The remaining non-BZ anxiolytics (buspirone, chlormezanone, hydroxyzine and meprobamate) are atypical in that they work through undefined mechanisms and have not been utilized or studied as widely as the BZ's. Meprobamate dates back to the pre-BZ era of the late 1950's but continues to be used today. Hydroxyzine has antihistaminic and sedative effects and is used for patients who should not receive BZ's. Chlormezanone has not been widely used in recent years and the newly developed drug, buspirone, has been utilized increasingly for anxiolytic therapy.

PHYSICAL DEPENDENCE POTENTIAL

Definition of Physical Dependence

Physical dependence has usually been defined in terms of the withdrawal syndrome observed upon cessation of chronic drug administration. Physical dependence is generally theorized to be a

TABLE 1:   Benzodiazepines and non-benzodiazepine compounds
           available for use as anxiolytics in the United States.

BENZODIAZEPINES APPROVED BY U.S. FDA	PRIMARY INDICATION
Slowly-Eliminated Desalkyl Metabolites	
Chlordiazepoxide (LIBRIUM)	Anxiolytic
Diazepam (VALIUM)	Anxiolytic
Flurazepam (DALMANE)	Hypnotic
Prodrugs for N-Desalkyl Metabolites	
Clorazepate (TRANXENE)	Anxiolytic
Halazepam (PAXIPAM)	Anxiolytic
Prazepam (CENTRAX)	Anxiolytic
Intermediate Elimination Profile	
Alprazolam (XANAX)	Anxiolytic
Clonazepam (CLONOPIN)	Anti-convulsant
Lorazepam (ATIVAN)	Anxiolytic
Oxazepam (SERAX)	Anxiolytic
Temazepam (RESTORIL)	Hypnotic
Rapid Elimination Profile	
Midazolam (VERSED)	Pre-Anesthetic
Triazolam (HALCION)	Hypnotic
NON-BENZODIAZEPINE ANXIOLYTICS	
Buspirone (BUSPAR)	Anxiolytic
Chlormezanone (TRANCOPAL)	Anxiolytic
Doxepin (ADAPIN, SINEQUAN)	Anti-depressant
Hydroxyzine (ATARAX, VISTARIL)	Anxiolytic
Imipramine (TOFRANIL)	Anti-depressant
Meprobamate (EQUANIL, MILTOWN)	Anxiolytic
Propranolol (INDERAL)	Anti-hypertensive

consequence of adaptative changes in drug-affected tissue systems which compensate for and produce tolerance to the direct effects of the drug.[2] Upon cessation of drug treatment, the withdrawal syndrome is thought to be an expression of these tissue changes manifested in the absence of the drug. There have been attempts to make definitions of drug dependence and withdrawal more functional by using the terms physiological dependence to describe physiological withdrawal signs and behavioral dependence to describe behavioral changes occurring as a consequence of drug abstinence. Whereas there may be merit in such functional distinctions, the current paper will consider physical dependence to be evidenced by a reliable withdrawal syndrome observed upon drug abstinence in individuals previously exposed to the drug. As such, the physical dependence withdrawal syndrome will be discussed as comprising the entire composite of all withdrawal symptoms and signs including physiological, subjective and behavioral changes which occur as a specific consequence of drug abstinence. Abstinence-related changes in drug-seeking and self-ingestive behaviors will be considered in the psychological dependence section and are not discussed as signs of physical dependence in this paper.

Physical Dependence Potential Assessed Outside of the Therapeutic Context

Physical dependence potential is usually assessed by one of three methods.[7] In *substitution tests*, physical dependence is induced by chronic treatment with a compound which is prototypic for the drug class under investigation and then the test drug is substituted to determine whether it will show sufficient cross-dependence to prevent withdrawal signs. The other two methods involve the chronic administration of the test compound in a dosage regimen that is known to produce physical dependence with the prototypic compounds. Subsequent to chronic treatment, signs of *spontaneous withdrawal* are evaluated following abrupt cessation of treatment and signs of *precipitated withdrawal* are evaluated following the administration of an antagonist which pharmacologically results in an abrupt cessation of receptor stimulation. In preclinical laboratory studies utilizing these methods, physical dependence has been shown to develop with many of the BZ's and barbiturates[7] but not with buspirone.[4] With BZ's and barbiturates, both the frequency and severity of withdrawal signs are generally thought to be increased by higher doses, longer duration treatment, and continuous rather than periodic treatment.[7,8]

Although early human laboratory studies systematically documented the parameters of physical dependence induction by barbiturate and non-barbiturate sedatives, only a few studies have examined physical dependence induction by BZ's in humans.[7,8,9] The first report of BZ-induced physical dependence in humans came from a study of eleven hospitalized psychiatric (mostly schizophrenic) patients who had been treated with high chlordiazepoxide doses (300-600 mg) for two to six months.[10] After abrupt placebo substitution under single-blind conditions, ten of the eleven patients showed symptoms and signs of withdrawal including depression, aggravation of psychoses, agitation, insomnia, nausea, anorexia and in two patients, grand mal seizures. These withdrawal signs developed 2-9 days following placebo substitution and were qualitatively similar to those observed with barbiturate and non-barbiturate sedatives.[9,10] Additional information has been obtained from a series of electrophysiologic sleep laboratory studies which have demonstrated rebound insomnia during the placebo washout period following short-term hypnotic use.[7,8] Following 7-14 days of nightly hypnotic administration in chronic insomniacs, double-blind placebo substitution produced rebound increases in wakefulness during the first three placebo nights following the quickly-eliminated BZ hypnotics, triazolam and midazolam, but not following the intermediate and slowly-eliminated BZ's, temazepam and flurazepam.[11] Although these sleep laboratory studies do not demonstrate classical sedative/hypnotic withdrawal symptoms, the observed rebound insomnia can be interpreted as withdrawal phenomena and may represent the early stages of physical dependence development.

Physical Dependence Potential Assessed Within the Therapeutic Context

For a long time, it was believed that physical dependence was difficult to achieve with BZ's and did not occur in normal therapeutic dosage regimens.[6,12] However, increasing numbers of reports identifying withdrawal difficulties in chronic BZ users have caused a re-evaluation of the physical dependence potential of BZ's. It is now well established that therapeutically-prescribed BZ treatment regimens can produce physical dependence.[1,12,13,14] Symptoms and signs which have been observed in chronically-treated patients withdrawn from BZ's include: anxiety, irritability, insomnia, dizziness, fatigue, confusion, sweating, nausea and dry retching, anorexia, dysphoria, headache, palpitations, tremor, muscle pains, muscle spasms and stiffness, depersonalization and derealization, perceptual disturbances including auditory, visual, gustatory and tactile distortions, paresthesias, feelings of motion, psychotic symptoms including paranoia, hallucinations and delusions, and finally, grand mal seizures and death.[1,12,14] Many of these withdrawal symptoms are similar to those produced by barbiturates and other sedative/hypnotics and therefore could be described as of the sedative/hypnotic type.

Based upon differences in severity and time-course, high dose and low dose benzodiazepine dependency syndromes have been suggested to be qualitatively and mechanistically different.[14] A high dose syndrome of the sedative/hypnotic type lasts for up to two weeks following abrupt withdrawal from high doses and a low dose syndrome shows a protracted time-course of less severe symptoms lasting weeks to months following discontinuation of normal therapeutic doses. However, it is not clear that high and low dose dependency syndromes represent different phenomena. Higher BZ dose users (e.g., 2-5 times normal therapeutic) are more likely to experience extreme withdrawal symptoms (e.g., delirium, seizures) after shorter courses of treatment (weeks to months) than are low dose users.[1,7,12] Many of the symptoms of low dose dependency are seen in both high and low dose users and seem to be minor manifestations of sedative/hypnotic withdrawal which follow a more protracted time-course than do the severe symptoms.[1,7,12] Symptoms most often observed in low therapeutic dose users resemble psychic and somatic manifestations of anxiety (e.g., anxiety, tremor, muscle spasms, anorexia, insomnia and faintness) and may be difficult to distinguish from symptom re-emergence.[12] However, the emergence of symptoms not previously experienced (e.g., tinnitus, headache, perceptual distortions) and transient rebound increases in previous anxiety symptoms suggest evidence of withdrawal phenomena which are not explained by a return of previous anxiety symptoms.[1,12] Additionally, even though low dose users are less likely to experience the more severe withdrawal symptoms, delirium and seizures have been observed in this population.[1] Overall, one can conclude that the probability and severity of a withdrawal syndrome is increased if: (1) higher doses have been taken; (2) on a chronic basis for more than four months; (3) the drug is stopped suddenly; and (4) a quickly-eliminated BZ has been used.[12]

There is still controversy over the prevalence of withdrawal phenonmena in therapeutic populations. Studies involving the withdrawal of self-selected patients seeking treatment for BZ dependence show a high incidence of withdrawal symptomatology approaching 100%.[12,15] Based upon a review of the world literature reporting cases of BZ dependence in the late 1970's, Marks estimated the prevalence of BZ dependence to be one case per 50 million patient months.[6] More recent studies involving controlled prospective and longitudinal observations have placed estimates in the range of one-third to one-half of all patients attempting withdrawal after at least four months of chronic treatment[1,3,12] and as many as 80% of patients withdrawn following more than 5 years of chronic treatment.[13,15] It is likely that these latter estimates are more realistic and have come to light now that BZ physical dependence is a recognized entity.

Patients physically dependent on BZ's usually are treated with a gradual dose reduction using a slowly-eliminated BZ such as diazepam[3,16,17] although phenobarbital has been advocated for this purpose.[14] Comparisons of abrupt placebo substitution versus gradual dose tapering with diazepam[17] have shown that abrupt dose termination results in a greater number and severity of symptoms and patient complaints but a less protracted time-course than occurs with the dose tapering. However, some patients may prefer a "cold turkey" approach which ensures a shorter course of withdrawal symptoms.[3] In order to avoid the development of physical dependence, good clinical practice currently recommends limited short-term BZ use on an as-needed basis with intermittent drug-free periods during which the need for continued pharmacotherapy can be evaluated or signs of physical dependence can be observed.[3] While intermittent use should reduce the likelihood or severity of physical dependence, a prospective withdrawal study suggested that even a history of discontinuous BZ use may sensitize patients to withdrawal effects as compared to patients without such histories.[15]

Comparative Physical Dependence Potential of Benzodiazepines

Much of the clinical literature on BZ dependence is based upon data from diazepam-treated patients; however, this is due to the greater prescription frequency of diazepam as compared to other BZ's. Increasingly, reports are citing cases of physical dependence on other BZ's.[6,13,16] There are two major pharmacokinetic factors thought to influence the degree of physical dependence and the severity of withdrawal symptoms.[7] Physical dependence is thought to develop as a function of the degree and continuity of receptor stimulation (i.e., dose × continuous duration). The severity of withdrawal is thought to be jointly determined by the degree of physical dependence and the rate at which drug receptor stimulation is terminated. Compared to the rapidly-eliminated BZ's, the slowly-eliminated compounds may be more likely to produce physical dependence (due to a more continuous exposure) but less likely to produce a withdrawal syndrome (due to the slow elimination of the drug which gradually weans the system from the drug).

Two prospective double-blind studies have suggested that BZ's with intermediate elimination profiles may produce more problematic withdrawal reactions than those with slowly-eliminated desalkyl metabolites. In patients with generalized anxiety disorder[13] who had received long term treatment with BZ's (83% > 3 yrs), those patients who previously received intermediate-elimination profile BZ's (i.e., lorazepam and alprazolam) showed more severe withdrawal symptoms on the first three days of placebo substitution and had higher drop-out rates than did those patients who previously had received slowly-eliminated BZ's (i.e., diazepam and clorazepate). However, there was no difference in the incidence of withdrawal symptoms (approximately 82%) between these two groups. In long-term BZ users attempting to gradually reduce their BZ dose,[17] an earlier onset of symptoms (1 day vs. 5 days, respectively) was observed in patients previously on intermediate-elimination BZ's (lorazepam and oxazepam) than in patients previously on slowly-eliminated BZ's (diazepam and flurazepam). Although there was only a non-significant tendency for their symptoms to be more severe, a greater proportion of the patients previously on the inter- mediate profile BZ's supplemented their withdrawal medication (actually placebo) with accessory BZ use than did those patients previously on the slowly-eliminated BZ's. Due to its rapid elimina- tion profile, triazolam has been suggested to have the highest de- pendence potential of all the BZ's.[18] Although sleep laboratory stud- ies have reported greater rebound insomnia with the rapid rather than the slowly-eliminated BZ's,[11] studies in laboratory animals have not supported the suggestion that triazolam has a greater po- tential for physical dependence than do other BZ's.[18]

Overall, these data support the conclusion that compared to the slowly-eliminated BZ's, more rapidly-eliminated BZ's produce a more rapid onset of symptoms upon abrupt withdrawal and that this rapid onset of symptoms may be perceived as more aversive. How- ever, it is not clear that this more rapid onset of initially more severe symptoms translates into a greater prevalence of withdrawal symp- toms or a measurably more severe syndrome at peak levels of with- drawal. There have been suggestions that compared to other BZ's, more problematic withdrawal reactions may occur with lorazepam[7] due to pharmacodynamic differences. However, until the data are more complete, one must assume that the individual BZ's cannot be qualitatively distinguished in terms of their potential to produce physical dependence.

Comparative Physical Dependence Potential of Non-Benzodiazepine Anxiolytics

Thus far in human[3] and animal[4] studies, buspirone appears not to produce physical dependence. Buspirone has been reported not to suppress the symptoms of BZ withdrawal in anxious patients[19] and a prospective study[15] reported BZ withdrawal symptoms following continuous clorazepate but not buspirone treatment for six months. Although a final verdict should await further experience with bus- pirone, these early data indicate that buspirone does not have the physical dependence potential of the BZ's and other anxiolytics. Early human laboratory studies of physical dependence with barbi- turate and non-barbiturate sedatives concluded that the chlordiaze- poxide withdrawal syndrome was slower to develop and more protracted than with barbiturates and meprobamate.[9] Systematic comparisons of the BZ's with barbiturates and meprobamate are lacking in the clinical literature although clinicians familiar with the use of these compounds often suggest that physical dependence and withdrawal problems are less prevalent and less severe with the BZ's.[6,8] Preclinical studies have suggested that spontaneous barbiturate withdrawal signs may be more severe than those produced by BZ's[8] although such observations may in part be due to pharmacokinetic differences in the rates of elimination of these drugs.[7] Overall, these data suggest that the physical dependence potential of barbiturates and meprobamate is as great and probably greater than that of the BZ's. Physical dependence phenomena with the other non-BZ anxiolytics have not been studied widely although physical dependence and withdrawal problems clearly do develop with these other drugs including antidepressants and beta-blockers.[2,3,5] With the interest in comparisons of BZ's and antidepressants, it is worth noting that several anti-depressant withdrawal symptoms resemble those seen in BZ withdrawal including "flu-like" gastro-intestinal disturbances, weakness, fatigue, headache, anxiety and sleep disturbances.[20]

PSYCHOLOGICAL DEPENDENCE POTENTIAL

Definition of Psychological Dependence

The World Health Organization has utilized the term, drug dependence, to encompass the psychic state which results from drug use and is characterized by a compulsion to self-ingest the drug in order to experience its psychic effects. Several of the DSM III-R criteria for substance dependence refer to chronic drug taking over which there is "impaired self-control." The term, psychological dependence, often has been used to describe the emotional craving for a drug. Therefore, the terms, dependence or psychological dependence, have been used ambiguously to describe both the cause and the effect of chronic drug ingestion and have been used as both descriptive and explanatory variables for the drug taking behavior pattern. Although there is no satisfactory definition of psychological dependence, it is clear that regular drug self-administration can occur in the absence of physical dependence[2,7] and that drugs which are not regularly abused may produce physical dependence.[2,3,5,7] Therefore, definitions of drug dependence must allow for the existence of drug self-ingestion behavior which can occur independently of physical dependence. It is reasonable to use the term, psychological dependence, to describe the existence of a reliable drug seeking or self-ingestion behavior pattern much like physical dependence is used to describe the existence of a pattern of withdrawal symptoms observed upon drug abstinence. As such, the term is used to describe the existence of a behavior pattern which could be considered "compulsive" but the term is not used as a causative variable to explain why that behavior pattern is observed. With this definition, psychological dependence is not synonymous with addiction since it does not necessarily involve the presence of deleterious consequences. Although this definition logically permits the existence of psychological dependence without physical dependence, it also allows the possibility that psychological dependence may occur as a consequence of physical dependence. A question to be addressed in this paper is whether there is evidence for a phenomenon involving compulsivity of drug self-ingestion and whether it occurs independently from or as a consequence of physical dependence.

Although there is no consensus on the causes of psychological dependence, the reinforcing effects of drugs are certainly one contributing factor. Therefore, the psychological dependence potential of anxiolytics can be assessed by examining the reinforcing effects of these drugs. The reinforcing effect of drugs refers to their ability to increase the probability of behavior resulting in drug administration (i.e., reinforce drug self-administration). Whereas abuse is distinguished from psychological dependence in that it involves less regular or compulsive drug self-ingestion, it is possible that drugs with a greater potential for abuse may also have a greater potential for psychological dependence. Therefore, studies assessing the likelihood of abuse may provide information on the psychological dependence potential of anxiolytics. In human studies assessing the abuse liability of anxiolytics, subject ratings of drug liking, positive mood or euphoria often are used to predict the probability of abuse with the assumption that these effects are factors contributing to the likelihood of drug self-ingestion and may be correlated with the reinforcing effects of drugs. However, suggestions that subjective effects of drugs are causally related to the reinforcing effects of drugs should not be assumed.[21,22]

Psychological Dependence Potential Assessed Outside of the Therapeutic Context

Several studies have demonstrated reinforcing effects of barbiturates and BZ's in drug self-administration experiments in humans and several animal species. A recent review of these studies[21] concluded that barbiturates and several BZ's reinforce drug self-administration behavior but that the BZ's do so less reliably than the barbiturates. It was also suggested that drug self-administration history may be an important factor influencing whether BZ's reinforce drug self-administration behavior. Human laboratory studies have shown that BZ's reinforce drug self-administration in subjects with histories of sedative abuse although they generally fail to do so in normal subjects without such histories.[8,22] The fact that BZ's are self-administered by non-physically dependent individuals from human and several animal species indicates that these drugs can serve as reinforcers in the absence of physical dependence; however, BZ's may be self-administered in a manner sufficient to induce physical dependence.[21] Whereas the presence of physical dependence has been suggested to enhance the reinforcing effects of drugs,[7] this has not been demonstrated for BZ's. Studies assessing subject ratings of drug effects have also reported that BZ's have a potential for abuse which is less than that of barbiturates and that subject ratings indicating potential for abuse are more consistently seen in subjects with histories of sedative abuse than in normal subjects.[22]

Two recent reviews on BZ's cited surveys of the general population and of drug abusing populations in order to estimate the prevalence of BZ abuse or psychological dependence in non-medical contexts.[7,8] Through the early 1980's, the prevalence of life-time recreational or non-prescription use of minor tranquilizers (mostly BZ's) reported by young adults and high school seniors has ranged from 11-15% and since the late 1970's has declined in a pattern corresponding to the decrease in the number of anxiolytic prescriptions nationally.[7,8] These lifetime prevalence rates are much less than those observed with other drugs of abuse (e.g., marijuana 59-64%).[7] Further analysis shows that recent use within the last month is much less prevalent (1.4%-2.1%) and regular or daily use is virtually non-existent.[8] Overall, these surveys of the general population suggest that BZ abuse is rare in the general population and that those who do abuse BZ's do so on an occasional and infrequent basis.[8]

In contrast to the low prevalence of abuse in the general population, observations from substance abuse treatment clinics indicate that BZ's and other anxiolytic/sedatives are abused. BZ abuse has been well documented in opioid abusers and methadone maintanence patients who may use illicitly-obtained BZ's to self-medicate other medical problems but who also use high BZ doses (usually diazepam) to "boost" the effects of the opioid.[7,8] There are regional differences between methadone maintenance clinics in the prevalence of BZ abuse, but estimates as high as 70% have been reported.[7] There are also high prevalences of BZ use in alcoholics although the majority of these patients report only prescription BZ use to treat anxiety or alcohol withdrawal symptoms.[8] In a survey of 163 patients being treated for BZ abuse or dependence,[23] 71 (44%) were considered mixed substance abusers who used a median of 40 mg (5-500 mg range) of diazepam (or equivalent) in combination with an average of 1.2 other drugs including: ethanol (47%); barbiturates (27%); opiates (27%); analgesics (27%); and cannabis (4%). Many of these mixed abusers initially used low BZ doses in a self-medication context but 48% reported patterns of dose-escalation, 37% reported an inability to stop due to withdrawal symptoms and the attending physician considered BZ's to be the primary drug of dependence in 32% of the individuals. In his 1978 review of the world literature reporting 477 cases of BZ dependence,[6] Marks attributed 401 cases to be in a mixed drug abuse context where BZ's were presumably obtained through "black market" sources and were used in combination with other drugs; only 99 of these 401 cases presented sufficient evidence to convince Marks that psychological dependence on BZ's was involved. Thus, although the prevalence is low, there are cases indicating primary abuse or psychological dependence upon BZ's outside of the normal therapeutic context.[6,23] However, most cases of BZ abuse are observed in "poly-drug abusers" who abuse BZ's in combination with other drugs and do so in an abusive pattern[6,7,8,23] probably not sufficient to be considered psychological dependence.

Psychological Dependence Potential Assessed Within the Therapeutic Context

The prevalence of psychological dependence upon BZ's in patient populations has been estimated to be extremely low based upon a variety of data.[8] Although data directly comparing barbiturates and BZ's are lacking, clinicians familiar with the use of these drugs suggest that patterns indicative of abuse, such as dose escalation and frequent prescription refills, have not occurred with the BZ's to the same extent as with barbiturate and non-barbiturate sedative/hypnotics.[5,6,12] Reviews of prescribing practice have concluded that BZ prescription patterns generally have been rational, cautious and appropriate.[5] Analysis of the patterns of prescription BZ use have also suggested that chronic, dose-escalating and compulsive drug taking patterns generally are not observed.[1,5,6,8,12] Indeed, many patients use BZ's only temporarily or in an intermittent manner corresponding to the occurrence of symptoms.[1,5]

Whereas the prevalence of psychological dependence on BZ's seems low based upon the above-mentioned data, some patients receiving prescription BZ's on a chronic basis apparently become psychologically dependent. There are reports of psychological dependence on BZ's in the absence of physical dependence as evidenced by the fact that some patients seemingly reliant upon their BZ medication may not show any detectable withdrawal symptoms upon final cessation of drug use.[1,6] In a review of the world literature reporting cases of BZ dependence through the late 1970's,[6] Marks identified 42 cases which reasonably indicated the development of BZ dependence within the therapeutic context. Of these cases, Marks identified 10 as displaying psychological dependence only, 12 as physical dependence only, 13 as displaying both physical and psychological dependence and the remaining 9 as of uncertain classification. Many reports have described patients who had difficulty withdrawing from BZ use despite repeated attempts to do so and despite their desire to reduce or terminate their prescription.[3,12,16] Clearly, many reports suggest that a major reason for difficulty in treating patients physically dependent on BZ's is the motivation of withdrawal avoidance which contributes to persistent BZ use.[3,16] Indeed, the frequency of recidivism or relapse to drug use following treatment-initiated drug abstinence suggests that psychological dependence may be strong in physically dependent patients. That recidivism is a problem with BZ's is illustrated by studies reporting on the treatment of patients who had failed in previous attempts to withdraw from medication.[13,16,19] Studies have reported that, following abrupt BZ withdrawal, 40-60% of the patients dropped out, were unable to complete withdrawal, or resorted to emergency supplemental BZ use to alleviate their withdrawal symptoms.[15,17,19] These data indicate that psychological dependence on BZ's occurs in the therapeutic context and that it may be particularly strong in cases of physical dependence.

Clearly, interpretation of psychological dependence is difficult in patients with chronic psychiatric illness. Since effective relief of anxiety symptoms is presumably dependent upon drug dose, it is entirely predictable that the chronically anxious patient would depend upon drug use for the "self-medication" of their symptoms. In anxious patients, who at one time terminated their BZ prescription use, as many as 80% have been observed to resume BZ use 6-12 months later due to a return of anxiety symptoms.[3,5] However, in a study of 50 regular benzodiazepine users who were treated for BZ dependence in a clinical pharmacology program, 70% had favorable outcomes in maintaining abstinence for 10 months to 3.5 years and only 14% showed poor outcomes or relapse.[16] The authors of this latter study suggested that their high success rate in maintaining abstinence may indicate that their patients had fewer chronic illnesses necessitating drug treatment. Although the situation involving a patient who depends upon BZ's for anxiety relief could still be considered a form of psychological dependence, society should not judge this to be addiction since the benefits of pharmacotherapy probably outweigh the risks of chronic drug use.

Comparative Psychological Dependence
Potential of Anxiolytics

Laboratory studies assessing the reinforcing effects of BZ's have consistently concluded that BZ's are less reinforcing than barbiturates but more reinforcing than drugs such as chlorpromazine.[8,21,22] Differences in the reinforcing effects of various BZ's have not been established.[21] Although rapidly-eliminated compounds such as triazolam and midazolam may produce higher rates of self-administration than do the slowly-eliminated compounds,[7,8] it is not clear that this indicates a greater reinforcing efficacy of these compounds. Based upon differences in the profiles of subjective effects, human abuse liability studies also have concluded that BZ's have a reduced potential for abuse as compared to barbiturates and methaqualone.[22] These studies also have suggested that BZ's having a slow onset of action such as the prodrug compound, halazepam, and the slowly absorbed compound, oxazepam, may have a reduced potential for abuse as compared to diazepam which has a very rapid onset.[7,22] Human studies of drug self-administration have also shown that diazepam was preferred over oxazepam in sedative abusers given a choice.[22] These laboratory-based predictions of lower abuse potential for oxazepam than for diazepam have been supported by epidemiological data indicating a lower incidence of abuse and abuse-related drug thefts for oxazepam which cannot be accounted for by differences in prescription rates.[7,22] Buspirone also may have a lower potential for abuse in comparison to diazepam. In rhesus monkeys buspirone was not self-administered[24] and in one human study, buspirone produced less euphoria than diazepam and produced more dysphoria at higher doses.[4,8] These data suggest that buspirone may not reinforce drug taking behavior and are consistent with one clinical report of higher dropout rates and more patient dissatisfaction with buspirone.[15] Because of concerns of abuse or psychological dependence, it has been suggested that patients with "addictive personalities" or histories of abuse who require anxiolytic medication should be given antihistamines or antidepressants instead of BZ's[3] since it is generally believed that these compounds have a lower abuse potential. In substance abuse treatment programs, clinicians often have noted the predominate use of diazepam among BZ abusers[8] and have suggested that diazepam may have a greater potential for abuse than other BZ's, possibly due to its rapid onset of effects.[12,22,23]

POTENTIAL FOR DELETERIOUS CONSEQUENCES

Definition of Deleterious Consequences

The delineation of deleterious consequences of drug use is an essential ingredient in the definition of drug abuse or drug addiction. Whereas the presence of physical dependence on a drug sometimes may be considered a deleterious consequence, this is not necessarily true since, in some cases, the disease state might be more debilitating than would physical dependence on the therapeutic agent.[5] Likewise, psychological dependence on a drug sometimes may be considered a deleterious consequence. Clearly with certain illicit drugs such as heroin and cocaine, drug seeking and drug taking behaviors may become so extreme that they interfere with other socially beneficial behaviors. However, depending on the pathology of drug-taking behavior, the development of psychological dependence may not be considered detrimental in and of itself. For example, even though some individuals may become psychologically dependent on caffeine, regular caffeine use is rarely indicted as socially impairing and many believe it is beneficial. Therefore, the development of physical and psychological dependence sometimes may be associated with deleterious consequences but this is not true necessarily. For these reasons, the three component characteristics of drug addiction (namely physical and psychological dependence and deleterious consequences) have received separate consideration in this paper.

Clearly the debilitating and sometimes life-threatening symptoms of sedative/hypnotic withdrawal may be injurious to the individual or to other members of society. Thus, physical dependence on BZ's certainly does have associated deleterious consequences and should be avoided by the use of intermittent rather than continuous BZ use if at all possible.[3] Whereas there is evidence of psychological dependence on BZ's and other anxiolytics in a medical context, the drug-taking behavior of patients who obtain their drug supply by legal prescription probably does not significantly interfere with other social behaviors. Although there are reports of psychological dependence on BZ's in a drug abuse context,[6] most illicit BZ use would be classified as abuse and not addiction. The remainder of this section will restrict itself to a discussion of the deleterious consequences of drug use other than those directly involving withdrawal symptoms or drug-taking behavior.

Deleterious Consequences Assessed Outside of the Therapeutic Context

The majority of experimental studies assessing deleterious consequences of drug use have involved measures of drug-induced deficits in human performance following single acute doses or short-term repeated drug administration in normal subjects. A review of this extensive literature is beyond the scope of this paper but virtually all of the BZ's, barbiturates, and non-barbiturate sedatives which have been tested have been reported to produce dose-related performance impairment on a variety of tasks presumed to measure different dimensions of human performance capability including perceptual, psychomotor, cognitive and memory dimensions.[8,25,26] The performance effects of antidepressants have not been widely studied so conclusions are limited but several antidepressants have been reported to impair psychomotor performance although possibly to a lesser degree than occurs with the BZ's and barbiturates.[25] Buspirone has been reported to produce very little or no psychomotor impairment at therapeutic doses or to produce relatively less impairment than BZ's at higher doses.[25] Whereas the majority of performance studies have been conducted in normal volunteers, similar performance deficits are seen in medication-free anxious patients following acute BZ doses[8] and in sedative abusers following the acute administration of BZ's and other barbiturate and non-barbiturate anxiolytics.[27] Studies of repeated dose administration in normal volunteers have shown that tolerance develops to the BZ-induced performance impairment but that the tolerance may be only partial or may develop at different rates with different performance measures.[8,28]

Deleterious Consequences Assessed
Within the Therapeutic Context

BZ's are clearly among the safest drugs ever developed. Many dermatological problems are associated with BZ and other anxiolytic use; however, these are not prevalent phenomena.[26] Clearly the greatest deleterious consequences of BZ and other anxiolytic use are those associated with CNS depression.[26] Epidemiological data as well as laboratory studies generally have suggested that BZ users are at increased risk of automobile and other types of accidents, although this risk is much less well defined than with alcohol.[8] Although sedation and psychomotor and memory performance impairment are to be expected with short term or intermittent BZ use, there is substantial tolerance to many of these effects during the initial phases of chronic therapy.[26] In anxious patients chronically using BZ's, sedation and psychomotor impairment generally are not observed although intellectual and memory impairments may be observed.[8,28] In anxious patients chronically using BZ's, short-term memory but not psychomotor impairments were observed in laboratory tests conducted following the administration of the patients' usual morning dosage.[28] Overall, these data indicate that patients receiving BZ's are at risk of suffering from performance impairment produced by these drugs and that cognitive or memory impairments may be more likely than are impairments of motor function. Fortunately, substantial tolerance develops to many of the adverse performance effects of BZ's so that patients maintained on lower doses are not as debilitated as simple extrapolation from the research laboratory studies might suggest. The few studies examining social adjustment of BZ users generally have not shown significant social impairments in chronic users.[8] There have been reports of BZ-induced increases in aggression and hostility; however, these effects are not prevalent and are probably idiosyncratic or more likely to occur in individuals with pre-existing aggressive tendencies.[8,28]

Comparative Deleterious Consequences
of Anxiolytics

The respiratory depressant effects of barbiturate and non-barbiturate sedatives which can cause death in overdose clearly make these drugs more dangerous than the BZ's.[5] Although BZ's may potentiate the effects of other CNS depressants, one can question whether any deaths have ever been caused by BZ's taken alone.[5] Whereas experimental studies of performance impairment have not documented differences between individual drugs consistently, there probably are meaningful differences which can be noted. Of the anxiolytics, buspirone may produce less impairment at lower doses[25] although higher doses have not been tested and further studies need to examine the nature of the impairments that have been observed before a final judgment is made. In subjects with histories of sedative abuse,[27] BZ's seem to produce relatively greater impairments of subjects' judgment and memory than barbiturates and non-barbiturate anxiolytics. With the nighttime use of BZ's as hypnotics, more slowly-eliminated BZ's are more likely to result in residual impairment on the next day than are the more rapidly-eliminated BZ's.[29] Although no study has directly compared different BZ's in a manner permitting definitive conclusions, there is reasonable evidence that the amnestic effects of triazolam are probably greater than with other hypnotics.[27,29] Whereas early reports of bizarre reactions to triazolam created a lot of controversy,[18] there are no reliable data suggesting that triazolam is unique in producing paradoxical psychotic reactions.[30] Compared to other hypnotics, there were greater numbers of reports of "adverse cognitive disturbances and psychotic symptoms" produced by triazolam in its first year on the U.S. market.[29] However, the meaning of these data is unclear since a variety of unrelated symptoms are apparently grouped together in this symptom category. For example, the most common symptom reported in this category was confusion which probably is related more to amnestic effects than to psychotic reactions.

GENERAL CONCLUSIONS

BZ's are undoubtedly among the safest drugs ever developed. Unfortunately, their relative efficacy and safety compared to the predecessor barbiturates permitted us to ignore their possible addiction potential. It is now well established that BZ's may produce physical dependence in chronic therapeutic dosage regimens. However, it is likely that intermittent dosage regimens involving BZ use on an as-needed basis will greatly reduce the incidence and prevalence of physical dependence in patient populations. BZ's have also been shown to produce psychological dependence. There is evidence suggesting that psychological dependence may be more likely in physically dependent patient populations; however, the chronic nature of anxiety disorders make clear definitions of psychological dependence difficult. The predominant deleterious consequences of BZ use are those related to physical dependence development or cognitive and psychomotor performance impairment. Whereas, pharmacokinetic differences between BZ's have been shown to produce predictable differences in the onset and duration of withdrawal phenomena in physically dependent individuals, available data do not suggest that there are reliable differences among the BZ's in their potential to produce physical dependence. Differences between individual BZ's with regard to their potential for psychological dependence or deleterious consequences have not been well demonstrated. The best available evidence suggests that slower onset BZ's such as oxazepam may have a reduced potential for abuse in comparison to rapid onset BZ's such as diazepam and that triazolam may have greater amnestic potential than do other BZ's. Compared to the predecessor barbiturate and other non-barbiturate sedatives, BZ's have a lesser potential to produce psychological dependence and do not produce respiratory depression and death. Of the available non-BZ anxiolytics, buspirone seems to have the lowest addiction potential; however, we should learn from history and be cautious before jumping on the buspirone bandwagon. Although meprobamate probably has an addiction potential similar to that of other barbiturate and non-barbiturate sedatives, studies comparing BZ's and meprobamate are generally lacking and it continues to be used today. Data regarding the addiction potential of chlormezanone and hydroxyzine are scarce and it is difficult to rank these compounds relative to the BZ's. Hydroxyzine is generally believed to have a lower abuse potential than the BZ's and sometimes is prescribed to addiction prone patients. While the antidepressants do produce physical dependence and a variety of adverse effects, their potential for abuse and performance impairment have not been widely studied and their clinical utility as anxiolytics remains to be determined.

REFERENCES

1. Petursson H and Lader MH. Benzodiazepine dependence. Br J Addict. 1981; 76:133-145.

2. Jaffe JH. Drug addiction and drug abuse. In: Gilman AG, Goodman LS, Rall TW and Murad R, eds. The Pharmacological Basis of Therapeutics, 7th ed. New York: Macmillan Publishing Co, 1985:532-581.

3. Rickels K and Schweizer EE. Current pharmacotherapy of anxiety and panic. In: Meltzer HY, ed. Psychopharmacology: The Third Generation of Progress. New York: Raven Press, 1987:1193-1203.

4. Ortiz A, Pohl R and Gershon S. Azaspirodecanediones in generalized anxiety disorder: Buspirone. J Affect Dis. 1987; 13:131-143.

5. Rickels K. Are benzodiazepines overused and abused? Br J Pharmac. 1981; 11:71S-83S.

6. Marks J. The Benzodiazepines: Use, overuse, misuse, abuse. Baltimore: University Park Press, 1978.

7. Griffiths RR and Sannerud CA. Abuse of and dependence on benzodiazepines and other anxiolytic/sedative drugs. In: Meltzer HY, ed. Psychopharmacology: The Third Generation of Progress, New York: Raven Press, 1987:1535-1541.

8. Woods JH, Katz JL and Winger G. Abuse liability of benzodiazepines. Pharmac Rev. 1987; 39:251-419.

9. Essig CF. Addiction to nonbarbiturate sedative and tranquilizing drugs. Clin Pharmacol Ther. 1964; 5:334-343.

10. Hollister LE, Motzenbecker FP and Degan RO. Withdrawal reactions from chlordiazepoxide ("Librium"). Psychopharmacologia, 1961; 2:63-68.

11. Kales A, Soldatos CR, Bixler EO and Kales JD. Rebound insomnia and rebound anxiety: A review. Pharmacology. 1983; 26:121-137.

12. Owen RT and Tyrer P. Benzodiazepine dependence: A review of the evidence. Drugs. 1983; 25:385-398.

13. Rickels K, Case WG, Schweizer EE, Swenson C and Fridman RB. Low-dose dependence in chronic benzodiazepine users: A preliminary report on 119 patients. Psychopharmacol Bull. 1986; 22:407-415.

14. Smith DE and Wesson DR. Benzodiazepine dependency syndromes. In:

Smith DE and Wesson DR, eds. The Benzodiazepines: Current standards for medical practice. Lancaster: MTP Press, 1985: 235-248.

15. Rickels K. Schweizer E, Csanalosi I, Case WG and Chung H. Long-term treatment of anxiety and risk of withdrawal. Arch Gen Psychiat. 1988; 45:444-450.

16. Aston H. Benzodiazepine withdrawal: Outcome in 50 patients. Br J Addict. 1987; 82:665-671.

17. Busto U, Sellers EM, Naranjo CA, Cappell H, Sanchez-Craig M and Sykora K. Withdrawal reaction after long-term therapeutic use of benzodiazepines. New Engl J Med. 1986; 315:854-859.

18. Griffiths RR, Lamb RJ, Ator NA, Roache, JD and Brady JV. Relative abuse liability of triazolam: Experimental assessment in animals and humans. Neurosci & Biobehav Rev. 1985; 9:133-151.

19. Lader M and Olajide D. A comparison of buspirone and placebo in relieving benzodiazepine withdrawal symptoms. J Clin Psychopharmacol. 1987; 7: 11-15.

20. Dilsaver SC and Greden JF. Antidepressant withdrawal phenomena. Biol Psychiat. 1984; 19:237-256.

21. Ator NA and Griffiths RR. Self-administration of barbiturates and benzodiazepines: A review. Pharmacol Biochem Behav. 1987; 27:391-398.

22. Griffiths RR and Roache JD. Abuse liability of benzodiazepines: A review of human studies evaluating subjective and/or reinforcing effects. In: Smith DE and Wesson DR, eds. The Benzodiazepines: Current Standards for Medical Practice, Lancaster: MTP Press Limited, 1985: 209-225.

23. Busto U, Sellers EM, Naranjo CA, Cappell HD, Sanchez-Craig M and Simpkins J. Patterns of benzodiazepine abuse and dependence. Br J Addict. 1986; 81:87-94.

24. Balster RL and Woolverton WL. Intravenous buspirone self-administration in rhesus monkeys. J Clin Psychiat. 1982; 43:34-37.

25. Smiley, A. Effects of minor tranquilizers and antidepressants on psychomotor performance. J Clin Psychiat. 1987; 48:(12, Suppl):22-28.

26. Edwards, JG. Adverse effects of antianxiety drugs. Drugs 1981; 22:495-514.

27. Roache JD and Griffiths RR. Lorazepam and meprobamate dose effects in humans: Behavioral effects and abuse liability. J Pharm Exp Therap. 1987; 243:978-988.

28. Lucki I, Rickels K and Geller AM. Chronic use of benzodiazepines and psychomotor and cognitive test performance. Psychopharmacology 1986; 88:426-433.

29. Bixler EO, Kales A, Brubaker BH and Kales JD. Adverse reactions to benzodiazepine hypnotics: Spontaneous reporting system. Pharmacology 1987; 35:286-300.

30. Lasanga L. The Halcion story: Trial by media. Lancet, 1980; 1:815-816.

Cannabis Dependence
and Tolerance Production

David R. Compton, PhD
William L. Dewey, PhD
Billy R. Martin, PhD

SUMMARY. The chronic abuse of many drugs produces both marked tolerance and physical dependence. Marked tolerance to cannabis has been observed in experimental animals and humans. However, reports of physical dependence, as characterized by significant withdrawal symptomatology upon cessation of chronic cannabis exposure, has not been well established or clearly defined in any species. The abuse potential of cannabis is more readily observed in humans than in experimental animal investigations. This may be due to the physiochemical characteristics of cannabis or Δ^9-THC, which complicates this type of animal experimentation. It is more likely that the greatest dangers of cannabis abuse involve the pharmacological effects of the drug upon the central nervous system and other organs, rather than the development of dependence.

Abuse of cannabis leaf (*Cannabis sativa L.*, known commonly as marihuana) has occurred for centuries. Ingestion of this material results in the absorption of many types of compounds, and of these the cannabinoid class has been the primary object of investigation

David R. Compton, William L. Dewey and Billy R. Martin are affiliated with the Department of Pharmacology and Toxicology, Medical College of Virginia, Virginia Commonwealth University, Richmond, VA 23298.

The authors would like to acknowledge the support of NIDA grants DA 03672 and DA 00490, and the Commonwealth of Virginia Center on Drug Abuse in the preparation of this manuscript.

Reprint requests may be addressed to David R. Compton, Department of Pharmacology and Toxicology, Box 613 MCV Station, Medical College of Virginia, Virginia Commonwealth University, Richmond, VA 23298-0613.

and interest. Essentially, of those cannabinoids which have been isolated, identified, and characterized, there are only four which have proven to be potentially important. They are Δ^9-THC (tetrahydrocannabinol) and Δ^8-THC, plus cannabidiol and cannabinol. Generally the pharmacological profiles of Δ^9-THC and Δ^8-THC are identical, though the Δ^9-isomer is about 1.5-3.0 times more potent in most cases. Cannabidiol and cannabinol have little or no psychotomimetic activity (euphoria, "high," alteration in mood or thought), but considerable evidence exists to suggest that either (or both) of these substances might contribute to the net effects produced by cannabis abuse, or possibly modify the direct pharmacological actions of Δ^9-THC. Recent reviews of the wide spectrum of pharmacological effects produced by cannabis or Δ^9-THC include those of Agurell et al.,[1] Dewey,[2] Hollister,[3] Martin,[4] and Razdan,[5] while potential therapeutic uses of cannabinoids (natural and synthetic) have been covered by Razdan and Howes,[6] and Mechoulam.[7]

It is important to note that a large number of cannabinoid analogs have been synthesized in attempts to identify which portion of the THC molecule is responsible for any one of the many effects produced by cannabis. Similarly, metabolites of Δ^9-THC plus many of the other ingredients found in cannabis have been isolated, identified, and synthesized in sufficient quantities to be studied in considerable detail. However, limited mention will be made in this chapter of the large numbers of cannabinoids in these latter categories. Few have been investigated for their abuse potential, and it is primarily cannabis abuse that is important in terms of the human condition. Thus, this chapter will be limited to the physical dependence liability and abuse potential of Δ^9-THC (the prototypical cannabinoid) and cannabis in humans and Δ^9-THC in laboratory animals. Reviews which are especially pertinent to the dependence and tolerance aspects of cannabis include those of Harris et al.,[8] Jones,[9] Kaymakcalan,[10,11] McMillan et al.,[12] and Wikler.[13]

DEPENDENCE IN ANIMALS

The most robust demonstration of physical dependence in laboratory animals has been in those cases where the drug to be given chronically possessed a very short half-life, or when an antagonist could be given to induce withdrawal. However, neither of these situations exist with the Δ^9-THC; therefore, it is very difficult to demonstrate physical dependence in laboratory animals. The long half-life and resultant long duration of action of Δ^9-THC is similar to that of the class of long-acting barbiturates. The long half-life of these drugs precludes the rapid induction of a drug-free system necessary for producing withdrawal. Generally, the chronic administration of a drug with a half-life of greater than 35 hours tends not to be followed by a withdrawal syndrome upon abrupt cessation of abuse.

Since Δ^9-THC has a very long half-life, it should not be necessary to administer drug every six hours (as is required for the opiates and other shorter acting drugs) in order to maintain a constant and sufficiently high blood level to produce tolerance or dependence-like phenomenon. Nevertheless, in monkeys, intravenous administration of Δ^9-THC every 6 hours, with increasingly larger doses for 14 days, and administration at the highest dose attained for 12 more days (36 day regimen) produced significant physiological effects during drug abstinence.[10] Symptoms appeared 12 hours after the last drug treatment, and continued for five days. Symptoms included anorexia, hyperirritability, aggressiveness, tremors and twitching, penile erection, and masturbation with ejaculation, as well as behaviors interpreted as hallucinations. However, it is not clear that the observed behaviors were in fact withdrawal, since Δ^9-THC was not clearly shown to reverse the effects. Similarly, after continuous intravenous infusion of Δ^9-THC (daily dose of 1.2 mg/kg) for 10 days, three of four monkeys suffered a disruption of schedule-controlled behavior.[14] Observers also noted that animals were aggressive and hyperactive during abstinence. Additionally, this withdrawal syndrome could be reversed by readministration of Δ^9-THC. These studies may indeed suggest that cannabis is capable of producing dependence in animals, though in either experiment the symptoms were not severe.

However, it has not been clearly shown that similar "withdrawal" symptoms may be reproduced in other laboratories, or using other routes of administration. It is possible that use of the intravenous route (uncommon in humans) produced a behavioral syndrome that cannot be observed with other routes of administration due to dosing limitations. An example of differential potency as a function of route is that intravenous Δ^9-THC produces antinociception equipotent to that of morphine (given either i.v. or s.c.), yet is 50-fold less potent by other routes.[15] Thus, the mild withdrawal syndrome observed in the monkey following intravenous administration may be unique to this route of administration.

Δ^9-THC produces a unique behavioral change in dogs first described as static ataxia by Walton et al.[16] The administration of effective doses of Δ^9-THC on a daily basis produced tolerance to this effect. Increasing the dose to very high levels did not overcome this tolerance. However, the administration of increasingly large doses of Δ^9-THC to dogs over 11 days did not produce withdrawal symptoms during an 8-day period of drug abstinence.[12]

Similarly to the situation in the dog, pigeons given daily intramuscular injections of very high doses of Δ^9-THC, up to and including 180 mg/kg, did not show withdrawal signs when the drug was removed.[12] Soon after the end of this treatment regimen there was a decrement in the operant behavior of the pigeons. However, this interruption of behavior was not felt to be an indication of withdrawal, since normal behavior was not reestablished when the drug was readministered.

Some authors have suggested that there are some common features between cannabis and opiates, and that certain actions of Δ^9-THC may be mediated by opioid related mechanisms in the central nervous system. A number of investigators have observed behavioral effects, which they have interpreted to be a withdrawal syndrome, due to chronic administration of cannabinoids followed by acute administration of a narcotic antagonist, such as naloxone. Tulunay et al.[17] reported that chlornaltrexamine (beta-CNA; a selective, long-acting irreversible opiate antagonist) inhibited the analgesia, hypothermia, and tolerance to hypothermia produced by Δ^9-THC in rats. Although there have been studies which have shown similar phenomenon, others have not been able to replicate these results.[14] Additionally, it is generally felt that this is not a true indication of withdrawal. First, there is no conclusive evidence indicating that naloxone specifically antagonizes acute cannabis behavioral effects, or that Δ^9-THC acts at the specific receptor site to which naloxone binds. Secondly, the effects observed are not reminiscent of the severity or type of withdrawal syndrome observed after cessation of chronic exposure to either the opiates or to other classes of drugs with long half-lives.

One type of substitution paradigm for ascertaining the possible dependence liability of the cannabinoids would be to determine if administration of Δ^9-THC prevented the withdrawal syndrome observed in an animal which had chronically received a different cannabinoid, an opiate, a barbiturate, or other dependence-producing substance. However, cannabinoids do not substitute for either opiates or barbiturates, thus showing that there is not cross-dependence between cannabinoids and opiates or barbiturates. These data suggest that even if physical dependence developed to the cannabinoids, there would not be cross-dependence with these other classes of drugs.

It is, of course, impossible to measure psychological dependence in laboratory animals. Self-administration of drugs may be an indication of psychological dependence and/or abuse potential (or craving). Yet, there are few reports which claim to have established experimental models where animals self-administer Δ^9-THC (or any of the majority of its analogs). The inability to maintain self-administration of Δ^9-THC was best shown when only a portion of the animals treated would self-administer Δ^9-THC after having had the drug administered to them for a long period of time prior to allowing the animal control of its drug supply.[10] In these experiments where animals had the opportunity to self-administer Δ^9-THC to prevent possible symptoms of withdrawal, only a small portion of the monkeys evaluated self-administered during the abstinence period. Instead, when given a choice, some monkeys self-administered cocaine rather than Δ^9-THC. This suggests that, even when experiments are designed to enhance Δ^9-THC self-administration, the abuse potential and possible development of psychological dependence to Δ^9-THC is tremendously less than to cocaine.

Another substitution technique which can be used to determine potential for abuse and/or psychological dependence is to use an animal that has learned to self-administer a baseline drug (cocaine, PCP), and determine whether the animal can be induced to acutely self-administer a different drug. Δ^9-THC (as well as related analogs) did not substitute for drugs with strong reinforcing properties.[18] This suggests limited potential for development of physical cross-dependence, as well as limited psychological dependence due to the weak reinforcing properties of Δ^9-THC. When animals cannot be trained to self-administer a drug, there is no other methodology available with which to predict psychic dependence in animals.

It is surprising that the cannabinoids, which produce a pronounced tolerance in laboratory animals (discussed below), do not show similarly severe signs of physical dependence. There are few other classes where such marked tolerance exists without the development of physical dependence. For instance, the level of tolerance developed to the cannabinoids far exceeds that observed with the barbiturates, which produce dependence with severe, life-threatening withdrawal symptoms upon abstinence.

TOLERANCE IN ANIMALS

For many psychoactive drugs, the development of dependence is generally associated with the production of tolerance. In fact the abstinence syndrome is sometimes easily described as a "rebound" response, or an exaggerated effect which is opposite of that produced by acute drug administration. This phenomenon can be attributed to drug-induced compensatory establishment of mechanisms to a different level of 'normal' activity in order to minimize acute drug effects. Additionally, the severity of the withdrawal syndrome is often a function of the degree of tolerance developed. Thus, consideration of drug tolerance is usually an important component in any discussion of withdrawal. However, this may not necessarily be the case with cannabis, since a tremendous degree of tolerance to Δ^9-THC can be observed, yet (as discussed) a similar degree of severity of symptomatology during withdrawal is not observed. This may, in part, be due to the unusually long half-life of Δ^9-THC, which is also an important factor to consider in those instances where tolerance develops after only a single administration of Δ^9-THC. Normally, sustained exposure of drug to the organism, tissue, receptor, etc. is required for tolerance development. Thus, either sustained release preparations or multiple daily treatments of a drug with a short half-life are required for tolerance development (cf. morphine tolerance). However, Δ^9-THC has a half-life estimated to be between 20-50 hours, with current results from Agurell and collaborators showing terminal phase elimination of 4.3 days. Thus single treatments of Δ^9-THC are somewhat analogous to multiple treatments of other drugs with relatively short half-lives (e.g., amphetamine, phencyclidine, morphine).

Specific cannabis-mediated effects to which tolerance develops, in a variety of species, can be found in other reviews.[8,9] Generally, tolerance develops to some degree to all cannabis-induced effects (provided proper procedures are used to examine the event). However, there are certain (apparent) exceptions, and in some cases the degree of tolerance development to particular effects is so slight as to be considered not of physiological importance.

Tolerance development has been shown to occur in all species studied. Parameters to which tolerance develops include simple physiological indices and complex behaviors mediated via the central nervous system. Some of these parameters in laboratory animals include Δ^9-THC-induced anticonvulsant activity, catalepsy, depression of locomotor activity, hypothermia, hypotension, immunosuppression, static ataxia in dogs, and alteration of response rates and accuracy on schedule-controlled behaviors.

The degree of tolerance that can be developed to Δ^9-THC is quite high. A 100-fold development of tolerance has clearly been observed in pigeons, dogs, and rodents. However, some reports actually indicate lack of activity with doses following chronic treatment which were 300- or 6000-fold higher than those initially effective in producing an effect. Tolerance has also been shown to the lethal effect of Δ^9-THC in pigeons; as a dose of 180 mg/kg, though inactive in tolerant animals, proved to be lethal in drug naive pigeons. Similarly, tolerance to the toxic effects of oral doses of Δ^9-THC as high as 250 mg/kg/day has been reported to develop in rats.

The onset of tolerance can be very rapid (1-2 administrations) or may not be observed until after a month of administration of drug four times per day. However, generally only 1 week of daily administration is required to observe tolerance to most simple parameters measured in rodents, dogs, or monkeys. Examples of tests showing rapid onset of tolerance include rodent hypothermia and decreased locomotor activity. In these cases a decrement in response can be observed 24-48 hours later upon administration of a second dose of Δ^9-THC, with nearly complete tolerance observed after a third treatment. In fact, after 6 daily administrations to rodents, a subsequent injection of Δ^9-THC produces an increase in body temperature rather than simple tolerance to the hypothermic effect. Since Δ^9-THC and related analogs have been shown to possess biphasic activity in some measures, it has been suggested that tolerance may develop to the sedative effects of Δ^9-THC, which allows the stimulant properties of Δ^9-THC to be observed. In the monkey, tolerance develops to the sedative properties of Δ^9-THC after two weeks of oral treatment, while tolerance to some excitatory components of behavior required two months of treatment prior to the development of tolerance. Thus, it is clear that tolerance develops differentially in all species as a function of the parameter measured.

Because of the noticeable differential rate in the development of tolerance to the effects of Δ^9-THC, some investigators have hypothesized the existence of an intriguing, almost subjective, component which may be involved in this phenomenon. In brief, tolerance is developed readily when the acute effect can be considered aversive, or detrimental to the subject. For instance, in a paradigm where the depressant actions of Δ^9-THC produced an increase in the number of shocks an animal received, then tolerance developed rapidly. In contrast, tolerance is developed slowly when the acute effect can be considered advantageous (if not actually desirable). For instance, in a paradigm where Δ^9-THC produced a decrease in the number of shocks an animal received, then tolerance developed slowly. Similarly, tolerance develops slowly (when at all) in those paradigms (discriminative stimulus) in which positive reinforcement (e.g., food pellets or water) is obtained following Δ^9-THC administration.

It is not necessary to treat animals daily in order to see development of tolerance. The drug administration interval of 7-9 days in the pigeon and 8 days in the dog has proven sufficient to maintain tolerance. Similarly one Δ^9-THC treatment per week, for a period of seven weeks, is sufficient to produce tolerance in pigeons to the suppressive effect of Δ^9-THC on response rate in positive reinforcement paradigms. Additionally, the tolerance developed using these kinds of treatment protocols is long-lasting. The tolerance development observed in the dog clearly was still present for at least 23 days. However, this does not always occur. Though tolerance may be observed for a period of months in some parameters, the tolerance developed to other effects of Δ^9-THC have been shown to last for only up to 24 hours.

Where tolerance has been demonstrated, there is no indication that the cause of tolerance can be explained based on alterations in pharmacokinetics. There is no evidence that the decreased effect of Δ^9-THC is due to an alteration in absorption, distribution, or metabolism. Thus, development of tolerance must be described as a pharmacodynamic event. This is meant to imply that there are compensatory (unknown) changes in central nervous system biochemistry and/or physiology responsible for the decreased effect of Δ^9-THC, as well as to include the possibility that there is a change in animal behavior due to learning within a conditioned state (behavioral tolerance).

There have been reports suggesting tolerance does not develop to some effects of Δ^9-THC. Prior to accepting this conclusion beyond the experimental conditions under which the data were generated, one should realize similar claims have not held true under more stringent testing criteria, or may not be relevant beyond the species and route of administration used. For example, in mice tolerance did not develop to the decreased locomotor activity effect of cannabis administered orally, yet tolerance did develop to intravenous Δ^9-THC. Additionally, tolerance was not observed to the effect of Δ^9-THC on body weight and food intake in rats in one study, yet was reported to occur in other studies. Tolerance is believed not to occur to the effect of Δ^9-THC on rat or rabbit EEG even after six daily treatments. In mice and hamsters tolerance does not develop to cannabis-induced depression of aggression. Additionally, tolerance does not develop in the dog to the anorexic or sedative effects of Δ^9-THC, or in the monkey to Δ^9-THC-mediated impairment upon intricate reinforcement schedule paradigms. However, in the case of these complicated behaviors, the question of state-dependent learning may play an important role in explaining the apparent lack of tolerance development.

DEPENDENCE IN HUMANS

It is well established that chronic heavy use of cannabis, or even hashish (oily resin of the cannabis plant with a higher concentration of Δ^9-THC), does not result in a withdrawal syndrome with severe symptomatology. The number of well controlled studies on the development of psychological or physical dependence to cannabis in humans is much less than those in various animal species. This may, at least in part, be due to the lack of identification of a good clinical use for Δ^9-THC, which would necessitate such studies. However, cannabis has been used for centuries, and there are a considerable number of reports in the literature regarding the long term, chronic use of this material. There is no evidence of anyone dying of withdrawal from Δ^9-THC, suggesting limited physical dependence. However, the occurrence of a psychological dependence, abuse liability, or craving is more probable than physical dependence. It has been difficult to draw conclusions from epidemiological data on the psychological dependence of marihuana given the plethora of social and legal factors that impact on the drug abuser. However, there are numerous case reports of psychological dependence to cannabis which have been reviewed by Jones.[9] Discontinued chronic use of marihuana results in symptomatology that has unique features for each case. However, in current society there are always questions as to why a user continuously seeks this class drugs. Does it merely result from a compulsive behavioral pattern that may or may not be directly related to the drug? Or is it merely peer pressure?

The early evidence for ''dependence'' upon cannabis arose from uncontrolled clinical observations following cessation of chronic drug intake. Most reports originated in countries such as India, Greece or Jamaica where cannabis or hashish had been used for long periods and was much higher in potency than the material smoked in the U.S.[9] Some of these reports provided a good description of the symptomatology that might be expected to ensue following abrupt cessation of prolonged use of hashish or cannabis, while other reports were merely little more that anecdotal. Regardless of their scientific merit, these reports serve to underscore the potential problems that could occur with constant exposure to cannabis. Fraser[19] reported that Indian ganja smokers who were suddenly deprived of cannabis became hyperirritable, experienced auditory and visual hallucinations, and masturbated incessantly for three to five weeks. Soueif[20] characterized abstinence symptoms in Egyptian hashish smokers as involving dysphoria, hyperirritability and insomnia. South African smokers reportedly experienced anxiety, restlessness, nausea, cramps, etc. when cannabis was suddenly unavailable.

Not too surprisingly, the conclusions reached by different investigators vary considerably, which is probably due to the vagaries associated with uncontrolled studies. However, there are some commonalities among the descriptions of cannabis withdrawal which include hyperirritability, tremors, sweating, auditory and visual hallucinations, dysphoria, anxiety, negativism, insomnia or abnormal sleep patterns. In reviewing case studies and animal experiments, Kaymakcalan[11] concluded smoking cannabis resulted in severe tolerance and dependence, and that the characteristics of cannabis tolerance were similar to those of opiate dependence. There are numerous problems with case studies which limit clear interpretation of these data. Most abusers do not restrict their drug use solely to marihuana. Frequently, in polydrug abuse, marihuana is used with drugs known to produce physical or psychological dependence, or are of high abuse potential (e.g., alcohol, stimulants, depressants). It is also well documented that some drug abusers also suffer from mental illness, and may be using illicit drugs for purposes of self-medication. The mental abberations that are sometimes reported during an abstinence period could be due to the reappearance of a mentally disturbed state as well as of drug withdrawal. For example, Knight[21] reported that one-fourth to one-third of male admissions to psychiatric hospitals in Jamaica had used cannabis. Of 74 males admitted to another psychiatric service over a 12-month period, 29 had used cannabis. Ten of these patients were diagnosed as "ganja psychosis," and four others were classified as "marijuana-modified mania."

Some of the symptoms of cannabis "withdrawal" that have been described in uncontrolled clinical studies have also been reported in more controlled experiments. In a very early study conducted by Williams et al.,[22] subjects smoked an average of 17 marihuana cigarettes daily for 39 days. Most of the subjects reported feeling "jittery" upon withdrawal, although observers were not able to detect any symptoms. Almost 20 years later, these studies were extended to Mendelson et al.[23] and Greenberg et al.[24] who placed subjects in a controlled environment and allowed them to smoke a self-determined number of marihuana cigarettes for a 21-day period. Upon termination of the smoking period, some subjects experienced rapid weight loss, decreased appetite, tremor, increased anxiety, hostility, decreased friendliness, etc. In a study with similar design to that of Mendelson and Williams, Cohen et al.[25] recruited volunteers to smoke marihuana for 64 days in a hospital. These subjects were allowed to self-medicate by smoking as many cigarettes as they wished, each containing 20 mg of Δ^9-THC. They smoked an average of 5 cigarettes per day between 4 and 12 p.m., the allowed self-medication period. Sleeplessness, anorexia, nausea and irritability developed after cessation of smoking. Georgotas and Zeidenberg[26] also allowed subjects to smoke marihuana cigarettes freely for a four week treatment period, which was preceded by a 10-day smoking period in which the marihuana consumption was increased gradually. During the first week of withdrawal the subjects became irritable, uncooperative, and experienced difficulties sleeping.

While similar conclusions can be drawn from the studies of Mendelson, Cohen, and Georgotas, there is good reason for cautious interpretation, as pointed out by Jones.[9] These studies lacked placebo or double-blind controls, and attempts were not made to reverse the withdrawal symptoms by reinitiation of marihuana smoking. Additionally, there are always problems with confining individuals for long periods of time. It may well be that some of the subjects exhibited mood changes as a consequence of confinement. It should be kept in mind that the subjects were aware of the treatment schedule, and therefore could anticipate termination of drug administration. The issue of self-medication has both advantages and disadvantages. Self-medication may well provide the most realistic treatment regimen for marihuana users, and therefore cessation of such treatment would have relevance to the real world situation. This treatment schedule allows the investigator to address the question "Does the pattern of marihuana smoking chosen by the user produce dependence?" On the other hand, self-medication can result in an uneven and erratic dosing schedule, with all subjects receiving a different dose. Thus, self-medication paradigms have serious drawbacks, and are probably inadequate for the investigator who is asking the question "Is it possible for dependence to develop to marihuana?"

Jones and his colleagues[9,27,28,29] studied the development of tolerance and dependence to cannabis and Δ^9-THC under a more rigorous treatment paradigm. It was assumed that if dependence did not result under these conditions, then it was highly unlikely that it would occur under less stringent conditions. The objectives of these experiments, in contrast to simply observing behavior following common abuse of marihuana, was to maintain high concentrations of Δ^9-THC in the subjects for long periods of time. To accomplish this, either Δ^9-THC or cannabis extract was administered orally to volunteers every three or four hours, 24 hours a day, for up to 21 days. Investigators chose to administer doses of either 10 or 30 mg of Δ^9-THC or the extract. The 30 mg dose of Δ^9-THC resulted in peak blood levels that were comparable to those obtained by smoking a marihuana cigarette. Cessation of treatment usually resulted in subjective effects which were first reported within five to six hours after the last dose of Δ^9-THC. The most prominent and frequent symptoms were increased irritability and restlessness. Other prominent and somewhat variable symptoms were insomnia, anorexia, increased sweating and mild nausea. Objective changes included body weight loss, increased body temperature, and hand tremor. Both the subjective and objective changes could be diminished by smoking a marihuana cigarette or by readministration of oral Δ^9-THC, suggesting establishment of a withdrawal syndrome. The intensity of the effects observed was dependent upon the length of the treatment time and the dose of Δ^9-THC.

It is not unexpected that the dependence phenomenon is directly associated with the amount and frequency of drug exposure. This causes some concern, since the Δ^9-THC content in marihuana has been rising for the past several years. As Wikler[13] cautioned earlier, the marihuana that has typically been smoked in the West has relatively low Δ^9-THC content (3%). Abuse potential, in terms of drug-seeking behavior, to low potency marihuana seems to be more a function of secondary reinforcement derived from the social situation in which marihuana is smoked, rather than a function of any pharmacological reinforcing properties of the drug. In cultures where smoking involves either marihuana of higher Δ^9-THC content (10%), hashish, or ganja, pharmacological reinforcement may play a greater role in maintaining substance abuse. While it is clear that the Δ^9-THC content of cannabis has risen dramatically above that which was smoked in the late 60's, it remains to be seen whether the concentration will continue to increase. Of course, it may be that the users will adjust their intake to compensate for increases in Δ^9-THC concentration. Alternately, this increased concentration may well lead to instances of development of physical dependence, though not one expected to be of very severe symptomatology.

TOLERANCE IN HUMANS

Most investigators suggest that pronounced tolerance must occur prior to the development of physical dependence to a drug. Clearly, Jones et al.[29] provided the most convincing evidence of tolerance development to Δ^9-THC in humans. Tolerance developed to cannabis-induced increases in cardiovascular and autonomic functions, to decreased intraocular pressure, to sleep disturbances and sleep EEG, as well as mood and behavioral changes in those subjects receiving oral Δ^9-THC.

It is not too surprising that there is less agreement with regard to the development of behavioral (i.e., psychic) tolerance to cannabis. Psychological effects can be highly complex and dependent upon many factors, not the least of which is the interaction between the subject and the environmental situation. It is also probable that the psychic effects produced by cannabis are mediated through several different mechanisms, and it would be expected that tolerance would not develop uniformly to all these mechanisms. It is a common characteristic among abused drugs that tolerance develops to different effects of a particular drug at different rates. This could be due to different effects being mediated by distinct types of receptors or second messenger systems in different brain regions. In the studies in which high doses of Δ^9-THC have been employed, behavioral tolerance has been found. For example, Jones[9] summarized studies with oral administration of Δ^9-THC in which tolerance developed to the subjective effects following a few days of 10 mg Δ^9-THC treatment administered several times each day. Ten days of treatment with repetitive 30 mg doses of Δ^9-THC produced even greater tolerance to the behavioral effects.

Tolerance to Δ^9-THC was best summarized by Hollister[3] who concluded that relatively little tolerance develops when the doses are small or infrequent and the drug exposure is of limited duration. Tolerance clearly develops when individuals are exposed to high doses for a sustained period of time.

CROSS-TOLERANCE

Since many classes of abused drugs produce euphoria (plus other similar effects), and since a large number of individuals are polydrug (not simply single drug) abusers, then the issue of cross-tolerance of cannabis or Δ^9-THC to other drugs is of considerable importance. The development of cross-tolerance between drugs could suggest that they share a common mechanism of action in instances where they produce similar pharmacological effects. It might be expected that drugs which exhibit cross-tolerance could be substituted for each other. There is little evidence for complete cross-tolerance between cannabis and other classes of drugs, which is consistent with the unique behavioral profile of the cannabinoids. Cross-tolerance did not develop between Δ^9-THC and the hallucinogens, such as LSD and mescaline in humans.[9] There are some suggestions of the existence of cross-tolerance between ethanol and Δ^9-THC, but the evidence is not strong. However, this does not imply there is no significant interaction when cannabis and ethanol are abused simultaneously. It does not appear that complete cross-tolerance develops between Δ^9-THC and any other drug of abuse. Additionally, cross-dependence has not been documented as a complicating problem with cannabis abuse. While it may be that some users addicted to other drugs will use cannabis to alleviate some of the symptoms during withdrawal, there is little evidence that cannabis will substitute for the primary drug.

INTERVENTION TREATMENT
FOR CHRONIC CANNABIS ABUSE

Although cannabis dependence is not a widespread problem, there are some individuals who become preoccupied with their abuse of cannabis. There have been efforts to provide assistance for individuals who have difficulty in stopping their marihuana use. Roffman and Barnhart[30] interviewed 225 individuals who responded to a public service announcement directed at adult chronic marihuana users. Seventy four percent of the callers reported that they were experiencing adverse consequences which were associated with their marihuana use rather than with other drugs, and 92% expressed an interest in being treated. Smith et al.[31] used a combination of aversion therapy with cannabinoid-free marihuana and self-management therapy to treat 22 volunteer chronic marihuana smokers for four weeks. These individuals significantly decreased their mean daily marihuana intake, prompting the investigators to conclude that this procedure offered promise as a treatment program for chronic marihuana smokers. There has not been, to the best of our knowledge, a follow-up evaluation of the problems associated with discontinuation of marihuana abuse in these volunteers. These studies demonstrate that there are segments of the population, although apparently quite small, that have difficulty controlling their abuse of cannabis, and will seek professional assistance.

CONCLUSIONS

Everyone grapples with the term addiction, particularly when it comes to quantification. Addiction in the simplest sense should be defined in terms of drug seeking behavior. There are many individuals who actively seek a continuous intake of either caffeine, nicotine, marihuana, cocaine, opioids, or many other drugs. There is good agreement that the consequences resulting from withdrawal (physical dependence) are quite different for each substance. Therefore, the real issue actually is the consequence of chronic use. Does abuse lead to physical dependence?

We have described the symptoms that have been reported when there is an interruption of the chronic use of marihuana or cessation of continual administration of Δ^9-THC to animals or humans. The relative intensity of the withdrawal syndrome is dependent upon the quantity (or dose) as well as the frequency and the duration of the use. Under the most intense exposure regimen, the symptoms of withdrawal are relatively mild in most subjects. If one considers the present existence of a large population of marihuana users, and the infrequent number of reports of medical problems following marihuana abstinence, then it is apparent that tolerance and dependence are not major issues. There are few reports in which the abrupt interruption in the use of marihuana has led to incapacitation of the individuals abusing this substance. The major issues of marihuana use are the direct effects of the drug, such as the effects on the reproductive system, immune system, lungs, etc.

It is important to point out that drawing the conclusion that marihuana is not a highly addicting substance does not sanction the use of this drug for recreational purposes. There is a small segment of the population that has sufficient difficulty controlling their abuse of cannabis that they seek professional treatment of the condition. Also, many individuals are polydrug, rather than single drug, abusers. Thus, abstinence symptoms due to cessation of chronic marihuana abuse may be masked by the continued intake of other euphorigenic drugs of greater abuse potential with concomitant severe withdrawal syndromes.

Of course, there are the special concerns with juveniles as to what effects marihuana use has on their physical, mental and social development. It should not be forgotten that, for obvious reasons, none of the clinical studies have been conducted with juveniles. However, anecdotal evidence does suggest that cannabis is detrimental to adolescent development. It is not known whether dependence and tolerance are more or less likely to occur in this young age population. The age factor has never been and never should be studied adequately to answer this question.

REFERENCES

1. Agurell S, Halldin M, Lindgren J, Ohlsson A, Widman M, Gillespie H, Hollister L. Pharmacokinetics and metabolism of other cannabinoids with emphasis on man. Pharmacol Rev 1986; 38: 21-43.

2. Dewey WL. Cannabinoid Pharmacology. Pharmacol Rev 1986; 38: 151-178.

3. Hollister LE. Health aspects of cannabis. Pharmacol Rev 1986; 38: 1-20.

4. Martin BR. Cellular effects of cannabinoids. Pharmacol Rev 1986; 38: 45-74.

5. Razdan RK. Structure-activity relationship in cannabinoids. Pharmacol Rev 1986; 38: 75-149.

6. Razdan RK, Howes JF. Drugs related to tetrahydrocannabinol. Med Res Rev 1983; 3: 119-146.

7. Mechoulam R. Cannabinoids as Therapeutic Agents. Boca Raton: CRC Press, Inc., 1986.

8. Harris LS, Dewey WL, Razdan RK. Cannabis—Its chemistry, pharmacology, and toxicology. In: Born GVR, Eichler O, Farah A, Welch AD, eds. Handbook of Experimental Pharmacology. Berlin: Springer-Verlag, 1977: 371-429.

9. Jones RT. Cannabis and Health Hazards. Toronto: Addiction Research Foundation, 1983: 617-689.

10. Kaymakcalan S. Tolerance to and dependence on cannabis. Bull Narc 1973; 25: 39-47.

11. Kaymakcalan S. The addictive potential of cannabis. Bull Narc 1981; 31: 21-31.

12. McMillan DE, Dewey WL, Harris LS. Characteristics of tetrahydrocannabinol tolerance. Ann NY Acad Sci 1971; 191: 83-99.

13. Wikler A. Aspects of tolerance to and dependence on cannabis. Ann NY Acad Sci 1976; 282: 126-147.

14. Beardsley PM, Balster RL, Harris LS. Dependence on tetrahydrocannabinol in rhesus monkeys. J Pharmacol Exp Ther 1986; 239: 311-319.

15. Martin BR. Characterization of the antinociceptive activity of intravenously administered delta-9-tetrahydrocannabinol in mice. In: Harvey DJ, ed. Marihuana '84, Proceeding of the Oxford Symposium on Cannabis. Oxford: IRL Press, 1985: 685-692.

16. Walton RP, Martin LF, Keller JH. The relative activity of various purified products obtained from American grown hashish. J Pharmacol Exp Ther 1938; 62: 239-251.

17. Tulunay FC, Ayhan IH, Portoghese PS, Takemori AE. Antagonism by chlornaltrexamine of some effects of Δ^9-tetrahydrocannabinol in rats. Eur J Pharmacol 1981; 70: 219-24.

18. Carney JM, Uwayday IM, Balster RL. Evaluation of a suspension system for intravenous self-administration studies with water-insoluble compounds in the Rhesus monkey. Pharmacol Biochem Behav 1977; 7: 357-364.

19. Fraser JD. Withdrawal symptoms in cannabis-indica addicts. 1949; 257: 747-748.

20. Soueif MI. Hashish consumption in Egypt, with special reference to psychosocial aspects. Bull Narc 1967; 19: 1-12.

21. Knight F. Role of cannabis in psychiatric disturbance. Ann NY Acad Sci 1976; 282: 64-71.

22. Williams EG, Himmelsbach CK, Wikler A, Ruble DC, Lloyd BJ Jr. Studies on marihuana and pyrahexyl compound. Public Health Rep 1946; 61: 1059-1083.

23. Mendelson JH, Babor TF, Kuehenle JC, Rossi AM, Berstein JG, Mello NK, Greenberg I. Behavioral and biologic aspects of marihuana use. Ann NY Acad Sci 1976; 282: 186-210.

24. Greenberg I, Mendelson JH, Kuehnle JC, Mello N, Babor TF. Psychiatric and behavioral observations of casual and heavy marijuana users in a controlled research setting. Ann NY Acad Sci 1976; 282: 72-84.

25. Cohen S, Lessin P, Hahn PM, Tyrell ED. A 94-day cannabis study. In: Braude MC, Szara S, eds. Pharmacology of Marihuana. New York: Raven Press, 1976: 621-626.

26. Georgotas A, Zeidenberg P. Observations on the effects of four weeks of heavy marihuana smoking on group interaction and individual behavior. Compr Psychiatry 1979; 20: 427-432.

27. Jones RT, Benowitz N. The 30-day-trip—Clinical studies of cannabis tolerance and dependence. In: Braude MC, Szara S, eds. Pharmacology of Marihuana. New York: Raven Press, 1976: 627-642.

28. Jones RT, Benowitz N, Bachman J. Clinical studies of cannabis tolerance and dependence. Ann NY Acad Sci 1976; 221-239.

29. Jones RT, Benowitz NL, Herning RI. Clinical relevance of cannabis tolerance and dependence. J Clin Pharmacol 1981; 21: 143S-152S.

30. Roffman RK, Barnhart R. Assessing need for marijuana dependence treatment through an anonymous telephone interview. Int J Addict 1987; 22: 639-651.

31. Smith JW, Schmeling G, Knowles PL. A Marijuana smoking cessation clinical trial utilizing THC-free marijuana, aversion therapy, and self-management counseling. J Subst Abuse Treat 1988; 5: 89-98.

Relative Addiction Potential of Major Centrally-Active Drugs and Drug Classes — Inhalants and Anesthetics

Trevor G. Pollard, MD

SUMMARY. The inhalation of a wide variety of substances for recreational purposes is a health problem of worldwide proportions. The inhalation of non-narcotic agents, such as volatile inhalants (e.g., solvents and glues), anesthetics and nitrites, adds significantly to the growing number of substance abusers. This is of particular concern because it affects the younger members of the population, and the substances abused are, for the most part, legally obtainable. The toxicity of these inhaled substances are reviewed and compared, as are their potentials for addiction and dependence.

INTRODUCTION

During the millenia-old quest for improved pain relief, experimentation with various substances has led to the discovery of many mind-altering drugs. The use of inhaled substances for recreational or mood-altering purposes has been recognized since ancient times.[1,2] The trances of the oracle of Delphi are hypothesized to have been carbon dioxide-induced. More recently, in the late eighteenth and nineteenth centuries, ether, chloroform and nitrous oxide (N_2O) were widely used for their euphoric effects.[3,4] As a social by-product of technological advancement, a wide variety of substances now exist whose inhaled vapors result in marked physiologic and

Trevor G. Pollard is Assistant Professor of Anesthesiology and Pediatrics, Department of Anesthesiology, University of Texas Health Science Center, 7703 Floyd Curl Drive, San Antonio, TX 78284-7838.

149

psychologic changes. In the early 1950's, the inhalation of the volatile fumes from a number of commercially available substances, usually solvents, was reported in the western United States. By the mid-1960's, this trend had swept the nation and spread shortly thereafter to western Europe.

While inhalation abuse is, for a variety of reasons, primarily a phenomenon of youth, adults are also involved. Although there is probably no limit to the experimental nature of humans and the wide variety of vapors available for intentional inhalation, recently developed classification schemes[2,5-8] lend some order to the more common of the seemingly disparate substances. For purposes of discussion, the three main groups of inhaled substances reviewed in this monograph will include the following:

a. volatile inhalants—a wide variety of volatile hydrocarbons, halogenated hydrocarbons, and other substances, excluding (b) and (c) below.
b. currently used anesthetics—both volatile and potent
c. nitrites

The epidemiology of the abuse of these substances and their toxicity will be reviewed, as will their addiction and dependence potentials.

INCIDENCE AND TOXICITY

Volatile Inhalants

The variety of substances abused by inhalation is quite remarkable. In most cases, the substance used is a mixture of chemicals in a volatile solvent designed for commercial or household use, such as adhesives/glues, cleaning and degreasing compounds, typewriter correction fluid, fuels (gasoline, kerosene, butane, diesel), antifreeze, and paint products. In addition, assorted aerosol products such as spray paints, deodorants, hair sprays, and food/cooking products have been used.[7] There has even been a report of asthma inhaler (salbutamol) abuse.[9] Usually it is the volatile solvents (alcohols, ketones, aromatic hydrocarbons) that produce the desired effects.

Widespread abuse of inhalants has been acknowledged since the mid-1950's. Subpopulations recognized since then as being at high risk include the young adolescent (predominantly male) from a low socioeconomic background with internal family stress[3,10,11] such as financial problems, parental alcoholism, and single parent families.[12] The age of abusers ranges from the child of four or five years to adulthood.[13,14] Inhalant abuse appears to be mainly a group practice, with frequency and duration of involvement ranging from a few times in one's lifetime to daily for years. The amount inhaled during one session varies widely.[15] In one study, lifetime prevalence for inhalant abuse in the adolescent was found to be as high as 16.5%[16] and daily use occurs in about 0.1% of the high risk group, compared to 6-10% for marijuana and 5-6% for ethanol.[2] Although usage tends to decrease with increasing age,[2] the current prevalence of inhalant abuse appears to be on the rise.[17]

The nervous system, both central and peripheral, is the primary organ adversely affected by the volatile inhalants. Most seem to cause a rapid disinhibition[15] (stimulation) of the central nervous system (CNS), resulting in a euphoric "high" which is undoubtedly the attraction that leads to the abuse of these agents. Concomitantly, there is drowsiness, gross and fine motor incoordination resulting in impaired locomotion and slurred speech, and occasional hallucinations.[15] There may also be an amnestic effect.[11] Other organ systems involved include the renal, gastrointestinal, cardiovascular, hematologic, musculoskeletal and pulmonary systems.

Because most of the substances inhaled are a complex mixture of solvents, it is frequently difficult to ascertain the molecular compound responsible for a given toxicity. Toluene was well-reviewed by McHugh,[2] and is one of the most common of these solvents, a component in adhesives and glues, acrylic paints, and thinners, all commonly inhaled substances. Its acute inhalation causes a central neuropathy characterized by an encephalopathy, resulting in behavioral changes (self-mutilation[18]), hallucinations, ataxia and convulsions. Chronic usage results in further CNS deterioration (neuropsychiatric disorders[19] and persistent cerebellar ataxia) as well as peripheral neurotoxicity. Although reflexes are normal, muscle weakness is noted, and rhabdomyolysis (rupture of muscle cells) is reflected in the raised serum creatine phosphokinase levels as high as twice normal.[20] This may be due to an indirect effect mediated by a neurotrophic dysfunction rather than a direct toxic effect, since certain muscles appear to be spared (central and respiratory groups).

Distal renal tubular acidosis has been noted in adults[19,20] resulting in severe electrolyte disturbances (hyperchloremia, hypokalemia and hypophosphatemia). Renal calculi, suspected to be due to increased renal excretion of hippurate,[19] a metabolite of toluene, have also been reported. These electrolyte abnormalities may also be responsible for the profound weakness. Complaints of nausea and vomiting, abdominal pain and hematemesis have been described in toluene abusers, ascribed to gastric irritation by benzoic acid, another toluene metabolite.[19] Although gastroscopy performed on 2/3 of these patients revealed no bleeding site, it is possible that a more distal bleeding site was present. Glue inhalation has also been implicated in severe vasospastic phenomena resulting in a right cerebral artery stroke, causing a dense hemiparesis[21] and a coronary artery spasm resulting in an anterior myocardial infarction.[22]

Gasoline has been shown to cause both peripheral and central nervous system toxicity, resulting in encephalopathy (seizures and EEG changes[3]), ataxia, tremor and myoclonus.[2] Some investigators ascribe much of gasoline's toxicity to the tetraethyl lead additives,[2,22] a theory which is supported by elevated serum lead levels[23] and improvement with chelation therapy.[2] Others think that N-hexane may be the toxic compound.[13] This theory is supported by the fact that naphtha, also containing N-hexane, has been shown to cause similar neuropathology, reflected in nerve conduction tests and biopsy studies.[24] Other adverse effects of gasoline sniffing include decreased appetite, weight loss, muscular weakness and cramps, as well as possible hepatic and renal damage.[3]

Halogenated hydrocarbons such as trichlorethylene, trichlorethane and bromochlorodifluoromethane are volatile agents commonly found in typewriter correction fluid and fire extinguishers.[2,25] The toxicity of this class of solvent is predominantly myocardial, very similar to halothane, a currently used anesthetic agent. These compounds are negative inotropes, causing significant direct myocardial depression, and resultant decreased cardiac output. There is a simultaneous sensitization of the myocardium to catecholamines resulting in increased generation of ectopic foci of electrical activity in the heart. This may result in ventricular fibrillation and death, a phenomenon referred to as "sudden sniffing death."[26] The danger of this may be increased during the act of breathing fumes from a plastic bag,[26] the most common mode of self-administration of inhalants, due to the increased arterial partial pressure of CO_2 caused by rebreathing. Other organ damage caused by halogenated hydrocarbons includes respiratory depression, hepatic necrosis and focal bleeding, and cerebrovascular accidents.[1]

As previously stated, determination of the toxicity of the separate constituents in these complex compounds has been quite difficult. Human studies would be all but impossible to conduct for obvious ethical and medicolegal reasons, and because the usual poly-drug use pattern of abusers would introduce excessive variability. Animal studies of pure solvent exposure have been criticized for dissimilarity to human exposure.[16] For these reasons, the actual components responsible for the toxicity of the halogenated hydrocarbons is still unknown.

Anesthetic Agents

Inhalation of the currently used anesthetic agents is a problem confined mostly to hospital personnel (operating room and emergency room technicians, nurses, anesthetists, surgeons and anesthesiologists),[27] presumably due to the lack of awareness by the general public of their existence, and to their relative inaccessibility. Nonetheless, in a recent review of 32 cases of N_2O abuse, nonmedical abusers included commercial suppliers of the gas, as well as industrial users.[4] N_2O is commonly used as a propellant in canned whipped cream, making this food product a readily available and legal source of an inhalant which produces a euphoric state. Also, the abuse of anesthetics stolen by members of the public has been recorded, including one presumed accidental death due to IV injection.[28,29] Although the incidence of chronic abuse appears to be low in comparison with similar abuse of narcotics and sedatives,[27] a recent survey of medical and dental students indicated that 20% had used anesthetic agents for recreational purposes.[30]

Inhalational abuse of the potent volatile anesthetic agents (halothane, methoxyflurane, enflurane, and isoflurane) appears less common while at the same time far more dangerous than the inhalation of N_2O. One review of potent anesthetic abuse revealed that 12 of 15 abusers of halothane died (some were suicides), and the only enflurane abuser also died.[27] Methoxyflurane abuse is quite rare,[31,32] especially in the United States where its use is limited mostly to veterinary anesthesia. The author was unable to find documented evidence of isoflurane abuse in the current literature.

The toxicity associated with the chronic abuse of currently used anesthetic agents is most completely described for N_2O. The most common manifestation of N_2O toxicity is a sensorimotor polyneuropathy, usually heralded by a tingling numbness of the extremities. This reversible process has been well studied, using nerve conduction velocities, somatosensory evoked potentials and visual brainstem evoked responses, all of which yield abnormal results.[33] Progression through continued abuse can lead to impotence,[34] ataxia secondary to sensory loss, recent memory loss and subacute delirium including visual hallucinations and paranoid delusions.[35,36] Bone marrow suppression has also been rarely associated with chronic N_2O abuse, leading to macrocytosis,[34,37] which may be linked to the inactivation of vitamin B_{12}, a crucial enzyme in the formation of the hematologic precursor, methionine.[37]

The toxicity of the potent anesthetic agents can be divided into acute and chronic. Acute effects, in addition to the sought-after CNS disinhibition, include respiratory and cardiovascular depression. To the abuser, the cardiovascular effects are of more concern; specifically, the myocardium is simultaneously depressed and sensitized to the irritating effects of catecholamines, as previously described for halogenated hydrocarbons. The effects of chronic exposure to these agents, well-known to the anesthesiologist, have been and still are being studied in relation to legitimate clinical exposure. They include hepatic and renal damage as well as possible suppression of the immune system. More recently, the worst of these effects, hepatic necrosis, has been described as a result of illicit use of these drugs.[27,31,32]

Nitrites

The use of volatile nitrites has been described since the mid-1800's, amyl nitrite being prescribed for its vasodilating properties to ameliorate the symptoms of coronary insufficiency. The use of amyl nitrite to enhance sexual pleasure became popular in the 1960's, particularly (but not solely) among the male homosexual community.[8,38] As a result, the federal government reinstituted a restricted status to the sale of amyl nitrite in 1969,[38] leading to the substitution of isobutyl nitrites, which are readily available in common unrestricted products such as room deodorizers. Recently, the popularity of nitrites among adolescent heterosexuals has increased, the purpose being to "get high" and escape the unpleasant realities of their day-to-day lives. Recent surveys of a high risk population (drug abuse treatment center residents) revealed a 43% lifetime prevalence of nitrite abuse, and at least 10% of those had used nitrites more than ten times[39]. In surveys of U.S. high school seniors, one survey showed that 10% had tried nitrites at least once, while another found that 8.6% of 3000 students had tried nitrites. Up to 0.5% of the group used nitrites on a daily basis.[40]

In 1980, the toxic effects of the illicit inhalation of nitrites was deemed "minimal,"[8] and included headache, nausea, and dizziness, all related to the marked vasodilation produced by nitrite inhalation. Two more recent comprehensive reviews of animal and human studies have pointed out an association of chronic nitrite abuse with the development of Kaposi's sarcoma, one of the hallmarks of acquired immunodeficiency syndrome (AIDS).[38,40] *In vitro* studies have revealed profound depression of human lymphocyte function by nitrites;[38] also, the metabolites of nitrites are N-nitroso compounds which are known to be highly carcinogenic in animals.[38] The results of a multivariate statistical analysis of AIDS patients was able to distinguish those patients with Kaposi's sarcoma from those with opportunistic infections, based on the patients' use of nitrites.[40] The results of these studies are controversial and have been challenged by conflicting reports; methodology has been criticized as the source of conflict, and there are ongoing human studies to determine the effects of amyl nitrites on immune function.[40]

Other toxic effects of inhaled nitrites involve the hematologic system. Methemoglobinemia has been reported from inhalation of butyl nitrite as has the occurrence of mild hemolysis in three patients, one of whom had G6PD deficiency. One case of massive hemolysis was reported in a patient with no known red blood cell defect, after inhalation of isobutyl nitrite.[41]

ADDICTION POTENTIAL

Volatile Inhalants

Although the chronic compulsive use of inhalants resulting in physiologic, psychologic or social harm, and the continued use of these substances despite the harm caused is simple to demonstrate, it is difficult to prove. Studies that attempt to determine addiction potential are frequently uncontrolled, often little more than a series of case reports. It is difficult to ascertain, for instance, that the social harm ascribed to gasoline abuse (e.g., violence, school problems) is not actually a manifestation of the poor socialization that led to substance abuse as a means of escape, rather than a direct effect of the inhalation. Most studies of the addictive potential of the volatile inhalants concern gasoline, toluene-containing substances and halogenated hydrocarbons.

Gasoline sniffers suffer not only the physical problems as previously outlined, but in addition develop social problems such as difficulties in school performance, social interaction (increased criminal activity, belligerent interaction with peers) and are at high risk for inadvertent thermal burns. Despite this, Watson reports a range of chronic abuse from once every few months to three or four times weekly.[12] In addition, gas sniffers seem to be at risk for recidivism after treatment, as seen in 11% of patients in one study, seen clinically for repeated sniffing.[42] It has been stated that the "sociological and psychological factors which motivate persons to become continuously intoxicated by gasoline vapors are the same factors which motivate persons to other forms of substance and drug abuse."[3]

Solvent (toluene) abuse is similarly addictive. Many case reports show repeated recidivism after several efforts to stop inhalation abuse, even while in a hospital setting,[14] sometimes severe enough to result in death[20]. Cohen has estimated that 20% of toluene abusers may become chronic sniffers.[43] Frequent users had significantly increased family, school, legal and peer-related problems.[10,44] In one study of 43 inhalant abusers, the majority used toluene and/or butane (50% for over one year), despite frequent demonic hallucinations which these patients described as fearful. When questioned, 92% regarded toluene as unsafe but enjoyable. The majority thought their lives would be shortened and their personal happiness decreased by inhaling toluene.[45]

Evidence that halogenated hydrocarbons (e.g., typewriter correction fluid) have addictive potential is weak. In fact, when interviewed, the residents of inpatient adolescent units denied any awareness of the harmfulness of their habit "other than passing out."[1] Nonetheless, one of the abusers had been comatose for ten days prior to return of normal function. One can only assume that the chronic use of these substances while denying obvious harm is indicative of an addictive potential.

It is clearly difficult to state unequivocally, based on sound scientifically controlled studies, that the volatile inhalants are addictive. In spite of obvious harmful effects of inhalational abuse, and well-documented chronic use, to strictly satisfy the definition of addiction as outlined in this monograph is problematic, simply because well-designed studies are lacking. Some investigators are of the opinion that sustained chronic use of inhalants is unusual, and that most abuse is transitory[46,47] and instigated by peer pressure, and that on the whole, physical and social problems rarely occur.[47] However, there is a small subset of inhalers (usually solitary sniffers[11]) in whom habituation can be expected, with accompanying physical and social problems. It is in this group that careful studies of addiction potential would be helpful.

Anesthetic Agents

Of the anesthetics, N_2O has been shown to have addictive potential. There is a reported naloxone-reversible interaction of N_2O as an agonist-antagonist with the mu, kappa and sigma opioid receptors in mice, which may help explain its addictive potential.[36] These are the same receptors that are implicated in the theories of human narcotic addiction phenomena. In a review of N_2O abuse cases, the majority of abusers exhibited addictive behavior.[4] N_2O has been used to substitute for ethanol, amphetamine and tranquilizer abuse by a patient who then developed neuropathic signs, which resolved on cessation of inhalation. Despite this resolution, he resumed his abuse with subsequent recurrence of the neuropathy.[36] As previously mentioned, professionals are often the abusers of this gas. Dentists have been identified as being at high risk for N_2O abuse, despite devastating personal, social and professional consequences.[48]

Although confirmed reports are sparse for the potent volatile anesthetics, it would appear that they, too, have addictive potential. More than one year of repeated use of halothane has been reported in a patient who routinely experienced vomiting and loss of consciousness as a result, and who eventually died from complications associated with pneumonia and hepatitis.[49] A similar effect has been noted for methoxyflurane,[50] inhaled repeatedly by an anesthesiologist during operative procedures for its mood-elevating effects, despite obvious judgment altering effects and physiologic side effects.

Nitrites

Volatile nitrites display addictive potential, although there is evidence that the potential is lower than the other inhalants. As previously described, there is widespread chronic abuse of nitrites by adolescents. Of 173 young adults in a drug treatment facility who were interviewed, at least 13% were chronic nitrite inhalers, yet the euphoric state achieved was described as "fair to good" by 56% and "not at all pleasant" by 44%.[39] Interestingly, the abuse of nitrites in homosexual men has decreased lately due to possible health-related problems outlined above.[40]

It would appear, then, that the volatile solvents, anesthetics and nitrites all have addictive potential since each group of substances is repeatedly abused by its own population of devotees in spite of well-documented, reproducible toxic side effects. It is impossible to conclude from the current literature whether the addiction is a physical dependence caused directly by the abused substance or a psychologic one, induced either by the euphoric state resulting from

CNS disinhibition or from the feeling of peer-acceptance. Volatile solvents seem to have the greatest addiction potential, followed by the anesthetics, then the nitrites. This impression may be artifactual, since incidence of solvent abuse is significantly greater than that of anesthetics or nitrites, with a proportionately larger case discussion in the literature, and since scientifically controlled studies are lacking.

DEPENDENCE POTENTIAL

Volatile Inhalants

The production of psychologic dependence on an inhaled substance, resulting in chronic abuse related to the reinforcing (rewarding) effects of that substance, is also an elusive point to scientifically prove. The rewards of substance inhalation vary from the thrill of experimentation and the peer-acceptance accompanying it, to the inexpensive avenue of escape from an unattractive reality.[47,51] Although studies specifically aimed at proving psychological dependence on volatile inhalants are few, there are frequent statements implying such dependence. Of 400 solvent inhalers in one review, 10% were thought to be psychologically dependent. Of those, all required professional assistance to stop their dependence, yet only one exhibited signs of physiologic dependence (see below). That author, however, stated that the division of dependence into psychological and physiological subgroups was of semantic interest only.[15] Another review of 43 solvent inhalers found that 92% of the inhalers found the process rewarding ("enjoyable") while at the same time 92% considered it unsafe, implying compulsion to abuse the solvent for its reward despite the known dangers[45]. With gasoline inhalation, the reward for continuous intoxication was the ability to face adverse life conditions — low socioeconomic status, and parental conflicts such as physical abuse and parental alcoholism.[3]

The production of physical dependence on volatile solvents, characterized by the development of tolerance and the emergence of withdrawal symptoms during abstinence, has been somewhat easier to document in the literature, probably due to the more concrete, objective measures used. Nonetheless, opinions concerning its development differ. While some investigators categorically state that physical dependence does not develop with solvents,[47] there are numerous citations, as early as 1962,[52] in which tolerance to glues,[15,52,53] toluene,[19,54] and butane[54] is well-described.

The evidence for the emergence of a withdrawal syndrome is less plentiful, and not quite as direct. Some authors think that withdrawal phenomena are either nonexistent (in the case of glue or gasoline abuse cessation),[12] or quite rare (1/400).[15] Others state that withdrawal symptoms are seen after chronic heavy abuse of solvents;[53] one study described withdrawal symptoms in 62% of patients who ceased toluene abuse and 50% of those who discontinued butane inhalation.[54] The symptoms were consistent with classic withdrawal from an addictive substance, including tremulousness, tachycardia, diaphoresis, cramps, agitation, disorientation, hallucinations, delusions, paresthesias and convulsions.[52-4] More indirectly, there appears to be some evidence that the solvents have been substituted for opioids by abusers, to avoid withdrawal, which may indicate some cross-habituation. All of 25 subjects in one study used toluene as an inexpensive and available alternative to heroin.[15] One poly-drug user substituted solvent inhalation for opioid use during an enforced in-hospital "drug-free" state, resuming his opioid abuse after discharge.[52] As no withdrawal symptoms were noted during this hospital stay, it may be that the solvent abuse ameliorated or prevented them, implying a cross-habituation and possibly supporting a physical dependence potential.

There is less discussion in the literature about physical dependence on gasoline. The consensus appears to be that withdrawal symptoms do not occur with cessation of gasoline inhalation.[3,12,47] The data on the development of tolerance is conflicting. Although the duration of each sniffing episode may increase,[3] the documentation of real tolerance remains difficult, perhaps due to the inability to quantitate the dose administered.

Anesthetic Agents

The inhalational abuse of anesthetic agents is rewarding due to their effects on the psyche. The majority of N_2O users found the sensations pleasurable[11,55] and up to 20% of medical/dental students have used N_2O in a group social setting for its euphoric effects.[56] Of the potent volatile agents, both halothane[49,57] and methoxyflurane have been sniffed as euphoriants, and halothane as a remedy for insomnia.[31] In addition, methoxyflurane was reported to enhance one anesthesiologist's ability to better tolerate an adversarial working relationship.[50] No reports of the psychological dependence potential of enflurane or isoflurane were available.

Physiologic dependence on these anesthetic agents, at least for NO, is an interesting problem. The evidence for the development of tolerance and signs of withdrawal is scant. Subacute toxic delirium has been reported after heavy chronic abuse of N_2O,[35] but it is unclear if the delirium was a toxic effect or a withdrawal symptom. However, a cross-habituation has been noted between N_2O and opioids, recently well-reviewed by Gillman,[36] in both human and animal studies. As with the volatile solvents (above), N_2O reduces opioid withdrawal symptoms[58] as well as ethanol withdrawal symptoms.[59] Although there is no evidence that the potent volatile anesthetics have physical dependence potential, there is no reason to suspect that they should be any different. It may be that the very high acute toxicity (lethal potential) of these agents, combined with the relative rarity of abuse, has so far prevented the discovery of their potential for physical dependence. Future animal studies may provide insight into this problem.

Nitrites

Finally, nitrites appear to be highly rewarding. They induce a perceived enhancement of sexual activity, specifically a more sensual and prolonged orgasm. In addition, among sexually promiscuous groups it has been touted as a social and sexual disinhibitor.[38] Many daily abusers of nitrites use them for their euphoriant rewards.[39,40] Thus, their psychologic dependence potential seems real. There are, however, no studies to date revealing a physical dependence potential of nitrites.

CONCLUSION

In summary, the abuse of inhaled substances is a worldwide health problem which until the past few decades had received little attention. The toxicity of these substances is now well-described in each of the different subset of inhalants — -volatile solvents and propellants, anesthetics and nitrites. Despite this, the practice of inhalation abuse is on the increase. Although the proposed reasons for this phenomenon are many and open to debate, the fact is that addiction potential for these substances is high. It is equally clear that a psychological dependence potential is present, although it is difficult to determine whether the dependence is due to the particular substance inhaled, to the act of inhalation, or to the social acceptance (perceived or real) one obtains through the act. Physical dependence on these substances should be easier to detect, due to the concrete nature of the signs and symptoms of withdrawal and the ability in most cases to quantitate intake, although as previously noted, the presence of withdrawal phenomena vary with the patient, the abused substance and the observing clinician. It has been only recently that efforts to determine a biochemical basis for dependence on these substances have borne fruit, in the case of N_2O; this is a fertile area for future research.

BIBLIOGRAPHY

1. Greer JE. Adolescent abuse of typewriter correction fluid. So Med J. 1984; 77:297-301.

2. McHugh MJ. The abuse of volatile substances. Pediatr Clin North Am. 1987; 34:333-40.

3. Poklis A, Burkett CD. Gasoline sniffing: a review. Clin Toxicol. 1977; 11:35-41.

4. Gillman MA. Nitrous oxide, an opioid addictive agent. Am J Med. 1986; 81:97-102.

5. Beauvais F, Oetting ER. Toward a clear definition of inhalant abuse. Int J Addict. 1987; 22:779-84.

6. Couri, D. Preclinical pharmacology and toxicology. In: Sharp CW and Brehm ML, eds. *Review of inhalants: from euphoria to dysfunction.* NIDA Research Monograph 15. DHHS Pub No (ADM)77-553. 1977; pp 98-101.

7. Domino, EF. Hallucinogens and inhalants. In: *Drug Abuse and Drug Abuse Research.* DHHS Pub No (ADM)87-1486. 1986; pp191-3.

8. Novak A, The Stash Staff. The deliberate inhalation of volatile substances. Journal of Psychedelic Drugs. 1980; 12:105-22.

9. Brennan PO. Inhaled salbutamol: a new form of drug abuse? Lancet. 1983; 2(8357):1030-1.

10. Reed BJ, May PA. Inhalant abuse and juvenile delinquency: a control study in Albuquerque, New Mexico. Int J Addict. 1984; 19:789-803.

11. Herzberg JL, Wolkind SN. Solvent sniffing in perspective. Br J Hosp Med. 1983; 29:72-6.

12. Watson JM. Solvent abuse by children and young adults: a review. Br J Addict. 1980; 75:27-36.

13. Hall DMB, Ramsey J, Schwartz MS, Dookun D. Neuropathy in petrol sniffer. Arch Dis Child. 1986; 61:900-01.

14. Davies B, Thorley A, O'Connor D. Progression of addiction careers in young adult solvent misusers. Br Med J. 1985; 290:109-10.

15. Watson JM. Solvent abuse: presentation and clinical diagnosis. Human Toxicol. 1982; 1:249-56.

16. Ron MA. Volatile substance abuse: a review of possible long-term neurological, intellectual and psychiatric sequelae. Br J Psychiatry. 1986; 148:235-46.

17. Osborn HH. Adolescent drug abuse: good news and bad. Hosp Phys. 1988; 24:13-18.

18. Gilmour AG, Craven CM, Chustecki AM. Self-mutilation under combined inferior dental block and solvent intoxication? Br Dent J. 1984; 156:438-9.

19. Streicher HZ, Oabow PA, Moss AH, Kono D, Kaehny WD. Syndromes of toluene sniffing in adults. Ann Intern Med. 1981; 94:758-62.

20. Lavoie FW, Dolan MC, Danzl DF, Barber RL. Recurrent resuscitation and 'no code' orders in a 27-year-old spray paint abuser. Ann Emerg Med. 1987; 16:1266-73.

21. Parker MJ, Tarlow MJ, Milne-Anderson J. Glue sniffing and cerebral infarction. Arch Dis Child. 1984; 59:675-7.

22. Cunningham SR, Dalzell GWN, McGirr P, Khan MM. Myocardial infarction and primary ventricular fibrillation after glue sniffing. Br Med J. 1987; 294:739-40.

23. Eastwell HD. Elevated lead levels in petrol "sniffers." Med J Aust. 1985; 143(Suppl):S63-4.

24. Tenenbein M, deGroot W, Rajani KR. Peripheral neuropathy following intentional inhalation of naptha fumes. Can Med Assoc J. 1984; 131:1077-9.

25. Steadman C, Dorrington LC, Kay P, Stephens H. Abuse of a fire-extinguishing agent and sudden death in adolescents. Med J Austr. 1984; 141:115-7.

26. Bass M. Sudden sniffing death. JAMA 1970; 212:2075-9.

27. Yamashita M, Matsuki A, Oyama T. Illicit use of modern volatile anaesthetics. Can Anaesth Soc J. 1984; 31:76-9.

28. Block S, Rosenblatt R. A halothane-abuse fatality. Anesthesiology. 1980; 52:624 (letter).

29. Berman P, Tattersall M. Self-poisoning with intravenous halothane. Lancet 1982; 1(8267):340.

30. Gravenstein JS, Kory WP, Marks RG. Drug abuse by anesthesia personnel. Anesth Analg. 1983; 62:467-72.

31. Okuno T, Takeda M, Horishi M, Okanoue T, Takino T. Hepatitis due to repeated inhalation of methoxyflurane in subanaesthetic concentrations. Can Anaesth Soc J 1985; 32:53-5.

32. Min K, Cain GD, Sabel JS, Gyorkey F. Methoxyflurane hepatitis. South Med J. 1977; 70:1363-4.

33. Heyer EJ, Simpson DM, Bodis-Wollner I, Diamond SP. Nitrous oxide: clinical and electrophysiologic investigation of neurologic complications. Neurology. 1986; 36:1618-22.

34. Blanco G, Peters HA. Myeloneuropathy and macrocytosis associated with nitrous oxide abuse. Arch Neurol. 1983; 40:416-8.

35. Sterman AB, Coyle PK. Subacute toxic delirium following nitrous oxide abuse. Arch Neurol. 1983; 40:446-7.

36. Gillman MA. Nitrous oxide, an opioid addictive agent. Am J Med. 1986; 81:97-102.

37. Nunn JF. Interaction of nitrous oxide and vitamin B12. Trends Pharm Sci. 1984; 5:225-7.

38. Newell CR, Adams SC, Mansell PWA, Hersh EM. Toxicity, immunosuppressive effects and carcinogenic potential of volatile nitrites: possible relationship to Kaposi's sarcoma. Pharmacotherapy. 1984; 4:284-91.

39. Schwartz RH, Peary P. Abuse of isobutyl nitrite inhalation (Rush) by adolescents. Clin Pediatr. 1986; 25:308-10.

40. Haverkos HW, Dougherty J. Health hazards of nitrite inhalants. Am J Med 1988; 84:479-82.

41. Bogart L, Bonsignore J, Carvalho A. Massive hemolysis following inhalation of volatile nitrites. Am J Hematol. 1986; 22:327-9.

42. Remington G, Hoffman BF. Gas sniffing as a form of substance abuse. Can J Psychiatry 1984; 29:31-5.

43. Cohen, S. The volatile solvents. Public Health Review. 1973; II: 185-214. In: Watson JM. Solvent abuse by children and young adults: a review. Br J Addict. 1980; 75:27-36.

44. Santos de Barona M, Simpson DD. Inhalant users in drug abuse prevention programs. Am J Drug Alcohol Abuse. 1984; 10:503-18.

45. Evans AC, Raistrick D. Patterns of use and related harm with toluene-based adhesives and butane gas. Br J Psychiat. 1987; 150:773-6.

46. Sourindrhin I. Solvent misuse. Br Med J. 1985; 290:94-5.

47. Masterton G. The management of solvent abuse. J Adolesc. 1979; 2: 65-76.

48. Aston R. Drug abuse. Its relationship to dental practice. Dent Clin North Am. 1984; 28:595-610.

49. Kaplan HG, Bakken J, Quadracci L, Schubach W. Hepatitis caused by halothane sniffing. Ann Intern Med. 1979; 90:797-8.

50. Perez de Francisco C. Pentrane Dependence: a case report. Brit J Psychiatry. 1971; 119:609-10.

51. Gilbert J. Deliberate metallic paint inhalation and cultural marginality: paint sniffing among acculturating central california youth. Addict Behav. 1983; 8:79-82.

52. Merry J, Zachariadis N. Addiction to glue sniffing. Br Med J. 1962; 2:1448.

53. Westermeyer J. The psychiatrist and solvent-inhalant abuse: recognition, assessment, and treatment. Am J Psychiatry. 1987; 144:903-7.

54. Evans AC, Raistrick D. Phenomenology of intoxication with toluene-based adhesives and butane gas. Br J Psychiatry. 1987; 150:769-73.

55. Atkinson RM, Green JD. Personality, prior drug use, and introspective experience during nitrous oxide intoxication. Int J Addict. 1983; 18:717-38.

56. Rosenberg H, Orkin FK, Springstead J. Abuse of nitrous oxide. Anesth Analg. 1979; 58:104-6.

57. Spencer JD, Raasch FO, Trefny FA. Halothane abuse in hospital personnel. JAMA. 1976; 235:1034-5.

58. Gillman MA, Lichtigfeld FJ. Analgesics nitrous oxide; adjunct to clonidine for opioid withdrawal. Am J Psychiatry. 1985; 142:784-5.

59. Gillman MA, Lichtigfeld FJ, Sandyk R. Subacute toxic delirium caused by nitrous oxide may be an acute withdrawal state. Arch Neurol. 1984; 41:704.

PCP and Hallucinogens

Marilyn E. Carroll, PhD

SUMMARY. In this review phencyclidine and related arylcyclo-hexylamines and hallucinogens, using LSD as the prototype, are considered as two distinct classes of abused drugs. Within these classes drugs that are found on the street are discussed, and a current epidemiological summary is provided. The abuse liability and dependence potential of these drugs are evaluated by considering four major determinants of their abuse. *First,* is the ability of a drug to function as a positive reinforcer and increase the probability of operant behavior leading to its delivery. Animal data describing the reinforcing effects of PCP are reviewed with respect to the influence of variables controlling drug-reinforced behavior; however, there are no animal models of hallucinogen-reinforced behavior. Several methods of quantifying reinforcing efficacy are discussed. A *second* determinant is the subjective effects of the respective drugs. These effects are described and compared across drugs based on clinical reports in humans and drug discrimination studies in animals. A *third* determinant is the behavioral and physiological toxicity that results from acute and chronic use of these drugs. Clinical reports and results of sensitive tests that have been developed for laboratory animals are reviewed. A *fourth* determinant is the dependence potential that exists with these drugs, measured by tolerance development and the extent to which behavioral and physiological disturbances occur when drug use is terminated.

DRUGS INCLUDED

Phencyclidine and its analogs are classified as dissociative anesthetics, a unique class of drugs that affects the central nervous system in ways that are different from hallucinogens. Initially PCP and related compounds were classified as hallucinogens like LSD. This

---

Marilyn E. Carroll is affiliated with the Psychiatry Department, University of Minnesota. Reprint requests may be sent to the author at the following address: Psychiatry Department, Box 392 UMHC, University of Minnesota, Medical School, Minneapolis, MN 55455.

167

was an inappropriate classification since hallucinations resulting from PCP use are rare and different in character from those produced by hallucinogenic drugs. In fact, PCP has been found to have a number of effects that are more like drugs in the sympathomimetic stimulants (e.g., amphetamine), CNS depressants (e.g., pentobarbital) and benzomorphan opioids than hallucinogens.[1] In this chapter phencyclidine (PCP) and related arylcyclohexylamines and hallucinogens will be discussed separately.

Only a small amount of experimental work was conducted with these drugs in the 1950's and 60's with human subjects. Subsequently, a number of legal constraints has eliminated the possibility for prospective clinical studies. While PCP and related arylcyclohexylamines are still classified by the DEA as schedule II (existing medical use and high abuse potential), there is no accepted medical use, and even production for veterinary use was terminated in the mid 1980's. The DEA classifies hallucinogens as Schedule I (no accepted medical use and high abuse potential).

As a result of the epidemic use of PCP which began in the late 1960's and peaked in the late 1970's, a considerable amount of behavioral and pharmacological research with animals has been funded by the National Institute on Drug Abuse. More data are available on the abuse liability and dependence potential of PCP and its related drugs than on LSD or any drug in the hallucinogen class; therefore, this review will be focused primarily on PCP and related drugs.

There are many PCP analogues with behavioral and pharmacological effects that are similar to PCP.[2] These analogues displace PCP from its receptor; they have similar effects on schedule-controlled and motor performance; they substitute for PCP as reinforcers;[2,3] and they share discriminative stimulus properties with PCP,[4-6] although potency differences have been noted. Other than a few studies investigating the potency, structure activity relationships and reinforcing efficacy of PCP and its analogues, most of the behavioral pharmacological research has centered on PCP. Furthermore, PCP analogues are only occasionally found on the street.

The hallucinogens have been classified into the following five groups according to their chemical structure: (1) lysergic acid amides (e.g., LSD), (2) phenylalkylamines (e.g., mescaline), (3) indolealkylamines (e.g., psilocybin), (4) other indolic derivatives (e.g., harmine) and (5) piperidyl benzilate esters (e.g., JB-329 ditran).[7] The first three groups will be considered together since their clinical effects have been reported to be virtually identical,[7] and animal studies show that they share discriminative stimulus effects.[8] Most of the information available on this group concerns LSD, the most potent drug in the group. Thus, the term hallucinogen, as used in the following text will generally refer to LSD, but it is assumed that the effects described would generalize to groups 2 and 3 (e.g., mescaline and psilocybin, respectively). Mescaline and psilocybin are rarely found on the street as are the drugs in groups 4 and 5 which are rarely used.

EPIDEMIOLOGICAL CONSIDERATIONS

In the most recent (1986) National Survey of American High School students and young adults it was reported that the lifetime prevalence (ever used) was 5% for PCP, 7% for LSD and 9.7% for other hallucinogens.[9] However, the percentages of use within the last year were 2.4% for PCP, 4.5% for LSD and 6% for other hallucinogens. Opiates, tranquilizers and sedatives were reported to be used less frequently in this population while cocaine, inhalants, stimulants, marijuana, cigarettes and alcohol were used more frequently. The usage rates for PCP and LSD have shown no increasing or decreasing trends over the last several years. The 1986 survey may currently be an underestimate as it does not reflect a recent upsurge in PCP use due to its combination with crack or cocaine base (space base). Increased use and toxicity from this mixture among a young adult population in Washington, D.C., Los Angeles and Miami has received considerable media attention in the last two years; however, prevalence trends for PCP and/or crack are not yet available for this time period.

DETERMINANTS OF ABUSE LIABILITY AND DEPENDENCE POTENTIAL

The purpose of this review is to discuss the addiction potential of PCP and the hallucinogens and to provide an estimate of their rank order with respect to a continuum ranging from least to most addicting. A comprehensive assessment of abuse liability and addiction potential would involve (1) the drugs' reinforcing effects, (2) subjective or discriminative stimulus effects, (3) behavioral and physiological manifestations of toxicity, and (4) behavioral and physiological changes related to tolerance and dependence. All four factors will be considered in an assessment of the abuse liability and dependence potential of each drug. *First*, a conceptual model that has been successfully used in both animal and human laboratory studies of alcohol and drug abuse is to view the drug as a reinforcer for operant behavior. A reinforcer is an event or consequence that is contingent upon a specific response and whose presentation increases the future probability of that response. The *second* factor is the subjective effects produced by the drugs. These can be measured by self-report in human studies or by drug discrimination studies in animals. For example, an animal can be trained to respond on one lever when a specific drug has been injected and another lever when saline or the vehicle has been injected. Generalization tests may then be conducted with a range of doses or different routes of administration to determine whether similar effects are produced. Drugs from other chemical classes may be compared, and cellular mechanisms of action may be explored by examining the stereospecificity of discriminative stimulus effects. The *third* factor to be considered as a determinant of abuse potential is toxicity. Drugs with minimal reinforcing effects and high potential for physiological and behavioral toxicity are considered to have high abuse liability (e.g., LSD) while others that have greater reinforcing effects but few disruptive features (e.g., caffeine) are not considered to have high abuse liability.[10] A *fourth* factor is the ability of a drug to produce tolerance and subsequently dependence measured by physical and behavioral withdrawal reactions when drug use is terminated. Although drug use is initiated and maintained in nondependent individuals, and animal studies have clearly shown that physical dependence is not a necessary condition for a drug to function as a reinforcer,[10] human drug users attribute relapse episodes to craving and other disturbances that occur during abstinence.[11] Furthermore, recent animal studies have shown more subtle and prolonged forms of withdrawal disturbances may occur after relatively brief drug exposure. These protracted effects may be a determinant of relapse.

ABUSE LIABILITY

PCP and Related Arylcyclohexylamines

Drug-Reinforced Behavior

Drug reinforced behavior has been distinguished from drug self-administration by a number of control procedures.[12] Criteria used in this review for drug-reinforced behavior are that behavior maintained by the drug exceeds behavior maintained by a vehicle, and the drug maintains orderly patterns of intermittently reinforced behavior. For instance, PCP has been demonstrated to function as a reinforcer by showing that responding diminishes when the vehicle alone is substituted for the drug.[1] Monkeys readily drink PCP solutions and prefer them to the vehicle (water) after only a few days or weeks of exposure. In addition, high rates of PCP-reinforced responding have been maintained by the use of second-order schedules.[13] In animal studies PCP has been shown to be a highly efficacious reinforcer. This is in sharp contrast to LSD and other hallucinogens. The reinforcing effectiveness of PCP in animals also conflicts with the relatively low rates of use in humans as revealed by survey and DAWN data. It is possible that PCP use is largely underreported because the population of users would not be reached in a survey of high school seniors, use of the drug does not often result in emergency room visits, and/or PCP is not always detected in blood or urine tests.

In addition to PCP, several arylcyclohexylamine analogues of PCP, compounds from the benzomorphan isoquinoline and dioxolane (dexoxadrol) classes as well as sigma opioid receptor agonists (N-allylnormetazocine) have been shown to function as reinforcers for primates and/or dogs.[1,14,17] It has also been demonstrated that these drugs share discriminative stimulus properties with PCP even when they don't appear to share reinforcing effects (e.g., cyclazocine).[1] Cross tolerance has also been demonstrated (Stafford et al., 1983), and one of these chemically dissimilar drugs (N-allylnormetazocine) has been shown to reverse behavioral disruptions occurring during PCP withdrawal.[14] These drugs are not currently abused, but their functional similarities may provide information about PCP's actions at the receptor level.

Variables Controlling Drug-Reinforcement

From clinical reports of human PCP users it appears that one variable that affects the self-administration rate is route of administration. The use of PCP in tablet form began in 1967, but PCP gained an unfavorable reputation, and its use nearly disappeared. In the early 1970's PCP reappeared as a substance that was sprinkled on marijuana and smoked, and by 1975 PCP had become one of the most frequently abused drugs. The use of PCP declined in the late 1970's and has remained stable as of a 1986 NIDA-sponsored survey.[9] Route of self-administration has also been shown to be an important variable in the animal studies. Intravenously delivered PCP has been established as a reinforcer in rats,[2] monkeys,[1] baboons[17] and dogs;[18] however, the intravenous route has been more difficult to establish in primates and leads to more toxic effects than the oral route. It has often been necessary to substitute PCP for a drug such as cocaine that is already functioning as a reinforcer. In contrast, orally-delivered PCP is rapidly established as a reinforcer for rhesus monkeys, but not for rats. Phencyclidine smoking has not yet been investigated in the laboratory.

Another variable that may determine PCP's abuse liability is its combination with other drugs and the changing prevalence of those drugs. Alcohol and marijuana are the drugs that PCP is often used with, and in the last two years there have been increasing media reports of users that smoke a combination of crack and PCP. The result, referred to as space base, may have the same potential as crack for increasing rates of compulsive use. Animal research has also revealed that when PCP is combined with barbiturates and alcohol in a number of species, the sedative effects of these drugs are enhanced.[1] One exception was in monkeys where low doses of pentobarbital increased behavior reinforced by orally-delivered PCP while high doses suppressed that behavior.[20] A similar biphasic effect was found with amphetamine.[20]

Dose is another variable that modifies PCP-reinforced behavior. Responding maintained by PCP and related drugs changes in an orderly inverted U-shaped function as drug dose or concentration is increased.[19] Drug intake (mg/kg) increases steadily as a function of dose except at the highest doses. This increase is less than that produced by ascending doses of opioids or barbiturates. Phencyclidine and like drugs have also been self-administered under a variety of reinforcement schedules ranging from those with low (e.g., fixed-interval) to high (fixed-ratio, progressive ratio and second order) response requirements.[2,13,17] Orally-delivered PCP can also maintain behavior under long interval schedules that delay the delivery of the drug for one hour or more.[21] This scheduling method allows responding reinforced by the drug to be unaffected by the intoxicating effects of the drug. Response rates as high as 156.6 responses per minute were maintained for an hour or more before the schedule allowed access to PCP. Since delivery of the drug depends on a minimal amount of responses after a specified elapsed time, high rates of responding may indicate greater reinforcing efficacy. This type of schedule has the potential for providing quantitative comparisons of abuse potential of different compounds within and between drug classes.

A variable that has recently been shown to have a marked effect on the reinforcing effects of PCP is the feeding condition. Food deprivation reliably increases PCP-reinforced behavior as it does with all other classes of drugs that are abused by humans.[19] The use of second-order schedules and fixed-interval schedules showed that response rates were markedly increased by food deprivation even when the amount of drug delivered at the end of the session was fixed. In contrast, the addition of an alternative drug (e.g., ethanol) or nondrug (e.g., saccharin) reinforcer reduced PCP-rewarded behavior. It has also been noted that changes in feeding conditions and alternative reinforcers are most effective at low and moderate PCP doses, but not at the highest doses.[22,23] These results suggest that the reinforcing efficacy of PCP and similar drugs are dependent upon the availability of other rewarding events in the environment.

Subjective Effects

Subjective effects or the feelings or mood states that are produced by a drug are an important factor in determining its abuse liability in humans. In animal studies drug discrimination procedures are used to determine whether the subjective effects of a drug are unique or whether they generalize to other drugs. The discriminative stimulus effects of PCP and other arylcyclohexylamines do not generalize to stimulants, depressants or hallucinogens, but they do generalize to some non-PCP-like drugs such as dioxolanes, benzomorphans and sigma receptor agonists.[24] Animal studies have also shown parallels in self-administration studies and drug discrimination studies with respect to PCP, its analogs, and these non PCP-like compounds.[2,25] The subjective effects of PCP in humans have not been studied in controlled laboratory settings by standard instruments such as the Addiction Research Center Inventory (ARCI) or Profile of Mood States (POMS) that are used to evaluate other drugs. Instead, our knowledge of these effects relies on retrospective reports resulting from surveys of PCP users.

Retrospective studies reveal two important effects of PCP. *First*, the subjective effects can vary dramatically depending upon the user's personality, and *second*, a user may experience vastly different reactions to PCP during different drug-taking episodes. In most cases low doses produce euphoria, feelings of unreality, distortions of time, space and body image and cognitive impairment. Higher doses produce restlessness, panic, disorientation, obsession with trivial matters, paranoia and fear of death. An interesting feature of PCP intoxication is that there is often amnesia beginning immediately after the drug is taken until the effects begin to wear off. These effects have been used to establish diminished capacity in some criminal trials involving PCP and correlated assaultive behavior.[26] Surveys indicate that the PCP experience is regarded as pleasant only about half the time and negative or aversive the rest of the time. Many chronic PCP users report that the unpredictability of the drug's effect is one of its attractive features.[27] The reports suggest that those who received a positive subjective experience from the first PCP use are more likely to develop a pattern of chronic abuse than those who initially experienced dysphoric effects.

Toxicity

The addiction potential of a drug may not only be determined by its positive reinforcing effects and other subjective effects. A comprehensive assessment of a drug's abuse liability would include its disruptive effects as well. In fact, a reinforcement-toxicity ratio has been discussed[10] as a means of comparing drugs and screening new compounds for abuse liability. The extent to which PCP intake may be limited (or enhanced) by acute effects that occur during and shortly after use of the drug as well as long term effects that may persist for more than 24 hours after substance use has ceased is not known. However, it has been shown that animals and humans continue to self-administer a drug even with experience or knowledge of its negative and/or toxic effects.

The acute effects of PCP and similarly acting arylcyclohexylamines (at moderate doses) begin within 5 minutes after the drug is inhaled or within an hour if taken orally, and they last up to 12-15 hours. The behavioral and physical symptoms vary according to dose and elapsed time after drug exposure. Physical changes after low doses are muscle rigidity, vertical and horizontal nystagmus, ataxia, increased liquid intake and urinary output and decreased pain sensitivity. After high doses, additional physiological symptoms include elevated blood pressure and heart rate, abnormal breathing, vomiting, convulsions and coma. Behavioral changes associated with lower doses are speech disturbances, rapid mood changes, agitation, belligerence, impaired judgment and paranoid thinking. Higher doses may also produce bizarre, violent or assaultive behavior, incoherent speech, blank stare, compulsive and repetitive movements and acute toxic psychosis.[27,28] There may be a sexual disparity in the violent behavior associated with PCP intoxication,[29] as it is seen much more commonly in males. Additionally there appear to be age differences in PCP's toxic effects. For instance, infants exposed *in utero* or young children receiving passive smoke exposure present with serious neurological symptoms such as stupor, seizures and coma. Psychotic behaviors are rare in children, and as in women, the combative features are usually absent.[30]

Long term effects of PCP have been more difficult to study in human subjects who do not often seek treatment and those who do enter the clinic typically have not been followed and tested after detoxification. However, existing studies indicate that chronic PCP use in adults does not currently appear to result in any measurable organ or cellular damage.[31] An analysis of clinical chemistries, electrocardiograms, chest x-rays and general physical examinations revealed no signs of toxicity in the liver, kidney or blood. In a recent study 6 rhesus monkeys that experienced up to 8 years of daily PCP self-administration (often accompanied by intoxication) were compared with 4 control monkeys that self-administered no drugs and 4 monkeys that had received sedative drugs for comparable periods of time. They were tested on 21 parameters of organ functioning, and they received complete physical examinations from a veterinarian specializing in primates. There was no indication of organic dysfunction (Carroll and Leary, unpublished data).

The form of long term PCP toxicity that is most damaging is the behavioral effects. In human users there are clinically defined mental syndromes associated with PCP use such as intoxication, delusional disorder or a mood disorder.[28] A delusional syndrome may emerge up to a week after PCP overdose. It is characterized by mild cognitive impairment, ritualistic, stereotyped behavior, dysphoric mood, rambling, incoherent speech and disheveled or eccentric appearance.[28] The mood disorder may emerge within one or two weeks after PCP use, and it is characterized by a prominent and persistently depressed, elevated or expansive mood featured by anxiety, irritability, somatic concerns, panic attacks, hallucinations and delusions. These disorders are not common, but they may be long lasting and suicide is possible. The physiological and behavioral effects of PCP intoxication described above also can lead to impaired social and occupational functioning.

The offspring of PCP users may be more at risk for long term behavioral toxicity in terms of prevalence and severity than adult users. In a study of 94 neonates with maternal PCP exposure and 94 controls, a significantly higher number of neurological abnormalities were reported in the drug exposed group including hypertonia and depressed neonatal reflexes than in the control group.[32] In a recent study of 12 PCP-exposed infants that were followed for 18 months there was no increase in congenital defects related to PCP use, but there was an unusually high percentage (67%) of medical problems (e.g., respiratory problems) during the perinatal period.[30] In many of the infants, irritability and hyperresponsivity continued for 6 months. Later evaluations indicated borderline to serious abnormalities in fine motor, adaptive, language and personal-social environment. These studies strongly suggest that developmental toxicity results from maternal PCP use.

Animal studies have provided a systematic and quantitative analysis of the behavioral effects of PCP and related arylcyclohexylamines.[24,27] Experiments with laboratory animals and PCP have shown that tests of performance, learning, memory and motor coordination is disrupted in a dose related manner after PCP administration. On tests of learning, PCP disrupts the acquisition process at doses that are too low to interfere with a well learned performance.[33] In this respect PCP is similar to d-amphetamine and pentobarbital but not MDMA, heroin and methadone. In a delayed matching to sample paradigm used to test memory in pigeons, PCP and pentobarbital, but not amphetamine and the opioids produced a similar disruptive effect.[24] The behavioral toxicity of PCP is further enhanced when it is combined with other drugs such as cocaine or amphetamine,[34,35] or CNS depressants.[36] In other studies PCP and THC decreased spontaneous motor activity in mice, and morphine enhanced a variety of pharmacological effects of PCP.[27]

Hallucinogens

Drug-Reinforced Behavior

Animal studies of hallucinogen self-administration are not found in the literature on reinforcing effects of drugs.[10,37,38] This is due to the failure to produce animal models of hallucinogen-reinforced behavior using intravenous drug substitution methods.[10,37]

Subjective Effects

Animal drug discrimination studies have indicated that hallucinogens are moderately discriminable as a distinct pharmacological class.[8,39] Drug discrimination studies have indicated that the discriminative stimulus effects of LSD are mediated by 5-HT receptors, as the LSD cues are diminished by 5-HT antagonists.[8] Furthermore, rats trained to discriminate LSD generalize to the indole (psilocybin) and phenylalkylamines (mescaline) and other 5-HT agonists but not to stimulants, sedatives, opiates and psychotomimetic and dysphoric agents such as PCP, ditran and cyclazocine.[8] The specificity of LSD, mescaline and psilocybin within the hallucinogenic class is unlike that of PCP which appears to overlap with other chemical classes.

The subjective effects of the hallucinogens in humans are derived from a minimal amount of experimental work and self-report case studies. In addition, there are elaborate accounts of hallucinogenic experiences in the popular literature of the 1960's and 70's. As with PCP, the subjective effects associated with hallucinogen use are strongly determined by a number of factors such as setting, expectations, user's personality, and dose. The experience is often euphoric; however, dysphoric features such as anxiety, depression, fear of permanent loss of sanity, paranoia and impaired judgment may exist. The most unique experience is the perceptual changes characterized by a sense of unreality, illusions, vivid visual hallucinations, synesthesias (e.g., "hearing colors" or "seeing sounds,"), distortions of body image, and infrequently, auditory and tactile hallucinations. One aspect of the hallucinogen experience that differs from that of PCP is greater alertness and clear memory for events taking place during the period of intoxication as well as the perceptual changes that were produced.

Toxicity

The onset of effects of hallucinogens is usually within an hour after oral ingestion, and the effects may last from 8-12 hours (e.g., LSD) to three days. Physiological changes can include: pupillary dilation, tachycardia, sweating, palpitations, blurred vision and incoordination. Flashbacks related to these perceptual changes are reported to occur in about 23% of regular users,[7] although it is not clear whether or not flashbacks are related to or predictive of dependence. The adverse psychiatric effects are the most damaging to normal social and occupational functioning. Three psychiatric disorders resulting from hallucinogen use have been described.[28] A *delusional disorder* may develop shortly after drug use and end within hours or turn into a long-term schizophreniform disorder. The prominent feature is persecutory delusions which may coexist with flashbacks. The *hallucinogen mood disorder* is similar to that described after PCP use. Depression or anxiety emerge shortly after drug use is terminated and may persist for more than 24 hours.

Suicide may be attempted. Finally, the *posthallucinogen perception disorder* is a more severe form of flashbacks. The symptoms usually last only a few seconds, but result in major depression, panic disorder and/or suicide. About half of the users that experience flashbacks experience a remission after several months, others experience them for years. Other forms of behavioral toxicity are homicide and self injury caused by impaired judgment (e.g., staring at the sun) and accidents (e.g., falls). There is no clear evidence of chromosomal damage to hallucinogen users or their offspring.[7] For instance a comparison of lymphocyte chromosomes in 57 Huichol Indians of Northern Mexico with multigenerational peyote (mescaline) use and 10 laboratory control subjects did not show a significantly higher occurrence of chromosome abnormalities in the Huichol Indian group that might be related to peyote use.[40]

There are currently few reports of simultaneous use of hallucinogens and other classes of abused drugs. A review of animal studies indicates that the effects of hallucinogens on operant or respondent (Pavlovian) behavior do not differ substantially from other psychoactive drugs.[8] One exception is hallucinogen-induced pausing that occurs with fixed-ratio schedules. This is a sensitive and specific test of the disruptive effects of hallucinogens.[8] There are also a few animal studies concerned with interactions of hallucinogens with other classes of drugs although they are not drugs that are abused. For instance, the effects of hallucinogens are mediated by drugs that alter serotonergic systems as well as those that affect opiate receptors.[8,41,42]

DEPENDENCE POTENTIAL

Phencyclidine

Tolerance

Tolerance to PCP and related arylcyclohexylamines has not been systematically investigated in humans, but chronic PCP users report that after regular use they increase the amount of PCP smoked by twice or more. Similar observations of tolerance have been noted in burn patients who require increased doses of ketamine.[27] Studies of tolerance using laboratory animals is typically conducted by changes in operant behavior before and during chronic administration of the drug. However motor coordination and stereotyped behavior have also shown evidence of tolerance development. The results of many animal studies indicate a 2-4 fold shift to the right in the dose-effect curve,[1] a relatively small amount of tolerance, compared to what other drugs produce. However, there are indications that continuous self-administration of PCP may lead to much greater tolerance development.[1] Animal research has also shown that tolerance is rapidly established and lost,[43] and this may account for the variability of acute effects in human users. Recent studies have attempted to determine whether tolerance is established by physiological mechanisms or whether the animals learn to behaviorally compensate for PCP induced disruptions. With one exception most studies indicate that pharmacological mechanisms such as biodispositional changes are involved.[1]

A recent study with rats indicates that supersensitivity, the opposite of tolerance, may also result from repeated administration of PCP.[44] The behavioral data and biochemical findings suggest that tolerance is mediated by the serotonergic neuronal system, specifically by down regulation of 5-HT$_2$ receptors, while supersensitivity is accounted for by increased mesolimbic dopaminergic neuronal function.[1,45]

Physical Manifestations of Dependence

Studies with laboratory animals reveal that chronic administration of PCP induces physical dependence after a relatively short period of chronic use.[1] In rats, abrupt withdrawal of i.v. PCP infusions after 7 days resulted in weight loss, piloerection, bruxism, susceptibility to audiogenic seizures and reduced exploratory behavior and motor (rotarod) performance. Withdrawal signs began at 4 hours, and dissipated within 24 hours of abstinence. Disrupted rotarod performance was also noted when PCP infusions were terminated after only 3.5 days of PCP exposure.[46] In rhesus monkeys intravenously-delivered PCP was self-administered for 50 days, resulting in marked intoxication and deteriorating health.[47] When saline was substituted for PCP, a withdrawal syndrome characterized by piloerection, tremors, irritability, preconvulsive activity, diarrhea, decreased food intake, bruxism and vocalizations was noted in all animals. The symptoms began within 4 to 8 hours after discontinuation of PCP self-administration, peaked at 12-16 hours and dissipated within 24-48 hours. In rats and monkeys the withdrawal syndrome was completely and immediately reversed by the acute administration of i.v. PCP.

Behavioral Manifestations of Dependence

The term behavioral dependence has been used to describe behavioral changes that occur during drug withdrawal.[48] This condition is contrasted with physiological dependence[49] which has been described as a stereotyped syndrome of physiological changes during drug withdrawal; however, behavioral and physiological dependence are considered different manifestations of the same process. The behavioral measures appear to be a more sensitive indicator of withdrawal than physical signs. Behavioral disruptions, usually defined by a change on an operant behavior baseline, are found during withdrawal from drugs that produce no physiological disturbances. They are also present with drugs that are capable of producing characteristic withdrawal syndromes at doses too low to produce those physiological changes.[50] Furthermore, behavioral disruptions often last several days after the physiological changes have cleared.

Recent laboratory studies have indicated that disruptions in behavior occur when PCP administration or self-administration is terminated. Slifer and coworkers[51] administered continuous intravenous infusions of PCP (0.05 mg/kg/hr) for at least 10 days to rhesus monkeys that had been trained to respond 100 times for the delivery of each food pellet. When a saline solution was substituted for PCP, food-maintained responding was markedly suppressed for 7-9 days. Mild physiological withdrawal signs were observed only during the first 24 hours of abstinence. This study was replicated in experiments with rats that received continuous intravenous infusions of PCP or its analog Ketamine for at least 10 days[52] or daily intraperitoneal injection of PCP for 7-10 days[53] and a similar protracted withdrawal disruption was obtained. In an experiment with rhesus monkeys in which PCP was orally self-administered and functioning as a reinforcer,[50] behavioral disruptions were noted up to 8 days after water was substituted for PCP. Reduction in PCP access to 1 or 3 hours per day or to 19.5 hours every 2nd or 4th day still resulted in reduced food-reinforced responding during PCP withdrawal.[50] In many of these behavioral studies the disruptions were rapidly reversed when PCP was readministered.[50-52] It is also noteworthy that in these studies the doses were relatively low and/or the access periods short such that little or no physiological disturbances were noted during drug withdrawal.

Clinical Reports

Although a PCP withdrawal syndrome is reliably produced in animal models by removing chronic drug access, a withdrawal syndrome in humans has not been clearly identified. For instance, the DSM-III-R[28] does not specify withdrawal symptoms from PCP and similarly acting arylcyclohexylamines as it does with other drugs such as opiates, sedatives and cocaine. However, there is increasing evidence from clinical reports of human PCP users and infants born to mothers that used PCP up to the time of birth that identifies a reliable set of withdrawal symptoms. A study conducted in 1981 with 68 chronic PCP users revealed that a third of this sample had sought treatment or medication to help them withdraw from PCP.[11] They reported symptoms of depression, drug craving, increased appetite, laziness and increased need for sleep. These symptoms usually occurred between one week and one month after termination of drug use. The lack of a clinically described withdrawal syndrome may be due to the fact that the drug is not taken in large enough quantities and/or not taken frequently enough to produce symptoms. Alternatively, the withdrawal syndrome may reliably occur in human users, but not be severe enough to bring users to a clinic.

Neonatal manifestations of maternal phencyclidine dependence have been easier to document than adult cases, and they occur quite reliably. Consecutive screening of 2000 pregnant women in a Cleveland, Ohio hospital between 1981 and 1982 showed that 7.3% had used PCP and 0.8% were verified current users by urine screening.[32] Initial case studies of the neonatal withdrawal syndrome described symptoms of irritability, hypertonic reflexes, diarrhea, poor feeding, inability to visually track, high pitched cry, and the infants were jittery.[30] In a recent study of 12 neonates exposed prenatally to PCP, all infants developed deviant neurobehavioral symptoms (e.g., irritability, tremors and hypertonicity) within the first 24 hours.[30] Symptomatic treatment with diazepam, phenobarbital or paregoric was administered for 2-12 days. The mean hospital stay was 8 days for the full-term infants contrasted with the average length of 2.5 days for full-term infants that were not withdrawing from drugs. The average hospital stay for the 5 preterm infants of PCP users in the sample was 24 days compared with 10 days for a nondrug control population.

Hallucinogens

Tolerance

Tolerance has been noted to develop rapidly to LSD, mescaline, DOM, and psilocybin but not to DMT and 5-MeODMT when the drugs were administered to rats and monkeys once per day.[54] However, tolerance did develop to the shorter acting hallucinogens DMT and 5-MeODMT when they were administered more frequently. Tolerance has been shown after repeated drug administration for 5 days in mice, 4 days in rabbits and 3 days in humans.[55] Similar rates of tolerance development have been shown in rats with bromolysergic acid, mescaline and psilocybin and in 7 days with humans. The extent of tolerance to LSD can be great as compared with PCP, ethanol, and other sedatives.[55] Cross tolerance has been demonstrated among LSD and indole and phenylalkylamine hallucinogens.[8] The order of potency found in animal studies and substantiated by human reports is that LSD is 10 times as potent as psilocybin and 100 times as potent as mescaline.[8]

Dependence

There is no available anecdotal or laboratory evidence of a withdrawal syndrome associated with termination of chronic hallucinogen use.

CONCLUSION

There are several ways to evaluate the relative abuse liability of PCP and specific hallucinogens. An epidemiological analysis among a young adult population would indicate the rank ordering is LSD, PCP and then other specific hallucinogens. These drugs as a whole would be ranked fairly low since most other drugs of abuse have higher prevalence rates (High School survey). Rankings take into account the current economic and social constraints, and they are probably not an accurate indicator of the drugs' inherent abuse liability and dependence potential. Thus, other assessments based on human self-report and laboratory animal studies need to be used.

Abuse liability and dependence potential are determined to differing extents by several aspects of the "addiction process." For instance, (1) the establishment and maintenance of drug-reinforced behavior, including the influence of variables (e.g., potency) that determine reinforcing effects, (2) subjective effects, (3) toxicity and (4) the extent to which tolerance and dependence are produced by characteristic patterns of self-administration. This comprehensive approach has been used in a systematic way to compare across drug classes,[10] but a formal comparison of PCP, its analogs and the hallucinogens has not yet been conducted. According to initial analyses PCP, TCP and PCPY are the most potent reinforcers of the arylcyclo-hexylamines and ketamine, PCM, PCE as well as several other PCP analogues show less reinforcing efficacy,[2,3,17,18] although the greatest difference in potency (e.g., PCP to ketamine) is only 5-10 fold. Further work is needed to adequately rank existing drugs as well as new compounds with regard to abuse liability and addiction potential. The following summary highlights the major areas where methods for quantification of drug effects are evolving.

Drug-Reinforced Behavior

There are several complex laboratory procedures that could be used to compare the reinforcing potential within and between drug classes. One method for comparing drugs as reinforcers is a choice procedure. The choice can either be exclusive (discrete trial) or concurrent. This method has generally been used to compare two doses or concentrations of a given drug, and the results from several studies indicate that higher doses are preferred to lower doses.[23] Another method would be to determine to what extent drug-reinforced behavior could be reduced by imposing a higher response cost[56] or an alternative reinforcer.[22] Again these methods have been used to compare different doses of the same drug, and results concur with choice studies; higher doses are more resistant to increased response cost or competing reinforcers. The progressive ratio schedule is a means of increasing response cost within a test session, and this method has been the one used most extensively to compare drug doses, across drugs within a class, and drugs in different classes. However, PCP and its analogs have been only partially studied,[2,10] and hallucinogens have not been evaluated in this way. In preliminary studies using these methods it was noted that phencyclidine analogs were not as potent as reinforcers as cocaine.[2]

Subjective Effects

Discriminative stimulus effects of PCP and the hallucinogens have been rigorously analyzed in animal research. For PCP-like drugs potency rankings have been noted for rats[6] and monkeys,[57] but there is disagreement across studies, and these potency rankings do not necessarily correspond with rankings of reinforcing effects.[2,3,17,18] There is some evidence that drugs that share discriminative stimulus effects are more likely to be substituted for the training drug and function as reinforcers than dissimilar drugs.[25,5,58] This connection should serve as a useful means of predicting abuse liability of newly developed compounds.

Toxicity

The behavioral toxicity of PCP analogues has been quantitatively described by a wide range of methods,[18] and PCP and its analogs fall on different parts of the toxicity continuum than they did on a continuum of reinforcing or discriminative stimulus effects. Thus, behavioral toxicity is a factor that should be developed as part of an overall assessment of abuse liability. As others have indicated, there are also subtle sensory and perceptual disturbances which may or may not accompany gross motor impairment as a result of drug use.[10]

Tolerance and Dependence

With respect to tolerance, PCP and its analogues have not been systematically compared, but PCP and LSD seem to both produce tolerance that is rapidly established and lost. Implications for the abuse of these drugs is that it may be difficult for users to regulate dose, a factor that may increase the abuse liability and dependence potential. Data from animal studies and human reports indicates physiological and behavioral manifestations of dependence for PCP but not for LSD. Thus, the relapse potential for PCP and related drugs may be greater than for that of the hallucinogens. Recent animal work with PCP,[50] THC[59] and cocaine[60] documents protracted behavioral disruptions that are rapidly reversed by administration of the drug. It is possible that these sensitive tests would reveal similar withdrawal disturbances when regular use of other drugs (e.g., LSD) is terminated; however, further work is needed to extend these methods to other drug classes. The importance of these findings for human users is that they may be at risk for relapse long after drug use has stopped.

REFERENCES

1. Balster RL. Clinical implications of behavioral pharmacology research on phencyclidine. In: Clouet DH, ed., Phencyclidine: An update. NIDA Research Monograph 64, Washington DC: Department of Health and Human Services, 1986; 148-162.

2. Marquis KL, Moreton JE. Animal models of intravenous phencyclidine self-administration. Pharmacol Biochem Behav 1987; 27:385-389.

3. Carroll ME. Oral self-administration of phencyclidine analogs by rhesus monkeys: conditioned taste and visual reinforcers. Psychopharmacology. 1982; 78:116-120.

4. Brady KT, Balster RL. Discriminative stimulus properties of phencyclidine and five analogues in the squirrel monkey. Pharmacol Biochem Behav. 1980; 14:213-218.

5. Overton DA. A comparison of the discriminable CNS effects of ketamine, phencyclidine and pentobarbital. Arch Int Pharmacodyn Ther. 1975; 215:180-189.

6. Shannon HE. Evaluation of phencyclidine analogs on the basis of their discriminative stimulus properties in the rat. J Pharmacol Exp Ther. 216:543-551, 1981.

7. Hollister LE. Effects of hallucinogens in humans. In: Jacobs BL, ed. Hal-

lucinogens: neurochemical, behavioral, and clinical perspectives. New York: Raven Press, 1984: 19-34.

8. Appel JB, Rosecrans, JA. Behavioral pharmacology of hallucinogens in animals: conditioning studies. In: Jacobs BL, ed. Hallucinogens: neurochemical, behavioral, and clinical perspectives. New York: Raven Press, 1984:77-94.

9. Johnston LD, O'Malley PM, Bachman JG. National trends in drug use and related factors among American high school students and young adults, 1975-1986. Washington, DC: Department of Health and Human Services, 1987; pp. 265.

10. Brady JV, Griffiths RR, Heinz RD, et al. Assessing drugs for abuse liability and dependence potential in laboratory primates. In: Bozarth MA, ed. Methods of assessing the reinforcing properties of abused drugs. New York: Springer-Verlag, 1987:45-85.

11. Tennant FS Jr, Rawson RA, McCann M. Withdrawal from chronic phencylidine dependence with desipramine. AM J Psychiatry. 1981; 138:845-847.

12. Meisch RA. Factors controlling drug-reinforced behavior. Pharmacol Biochem Behav. 1987; 27:367-371.

13. Meisch RA, Carroll ME. Oral drug self-administration: drugs as reinforcers. In: Bozarth MA, ed. Methods of assessing the reinforcing properties of abused drugs. New York: Springer-Verlag, 1987; 143-160.

14. Carroll ME. Oral self-administration of N-allylnormetazocine (SKF-10,047) stereoisomers in rhesus monkeys: substitution during phencyclidine self-administration and withdrawal. Pharmacol Biochem Behav. 1988; 30:493-500.

15. Vaupel DB, Risner ME, Shannon HE. Pharmacologic and reinforcing properties of phencyclidine and the enantiomers of N-allynormetazocine in the dog. Dr. Alc Dep 1986; 18:173-194.

16. Stafford I, Tomie A, Wagner GC. Effects of SKF-10047 in the phencyclidine-dependent rat: evidence for common receptor mechanisms. Dr. Dep. 1983; 12:151-156.

17. Lukas SE, Griffiths RR, Brady JV, et al. Phencyclidine-analogue self-injection by the baboon. Psychopharmacology, 1984; 83:316-320.

18. Risner ME. Intravenous self-administration of phencyclidine and related compounds in the dog. J Pharmacol Exp Ther. 1982; 221:637-644.

19. Carroll ME, Meisch RA. Increased drug-reinforced behavior due to food deprivation. In: Thompson T, Dews PB, Barrett JE, eds. Advances in behavioral pharmacology, Vol. 4. New York: Academic Press, 1984: 779-787.

20. Carroll ME. Effects of pentobarbital and d-amphetamine on oral phencyclidine self-administration in rhesus monkeys. Pharmacol Biochem Behav. 1984; 20:137-143.

21. Carroll ME. Performance maintained by orally-delivered phencyclidine under second-order, tandem and fixed-interval schedules in food-satiated and food-deprived rhesus monkeys. J Pharmacol Exp Ther. 1985; 232:351-359.

22. Carroll ME. Concurrent phencyclidine and saccharin access: presentation of an alternative reinforcer reduces drug intake. J Exp Anal Behav. 1985; 4;131-144.

23. Carroll, ME. Concurrent access to two concentrations of orally-delivered phencyclidine: effects of feeding conditions. J Exp Anal Behav. 1987; 47:347-362.

24. Balster RL. The behavioral pharmacology of phencyclidine. Psychopharmacology: the third generation of progress. New York: Raven Press, 1987:1573-1579.

25. Young AM, Herling S, Winger GD et al. Comparison of discriminative and reinforcing effects of ketamine and related compounds in the rhesus monkey. NIDA Research Monograph 34. DHHS Pub. No. (ADM) 81-1058. Washington DC: Sept, DOC., U.S. Govt. Print. Off. 1981; 173-179.

26. Siegel RK. Phencyclidine, criminal behavior, and the defense of diminished capacity. In: Peterson RC, Stillman RC, ed. Phencyclidine (PCP) abuse: an appraisal. Washington, DC.: Department of Health and Human Services; 1978, 272-288.

27. Carroll ME. PCP the dangerous angel. In: Snyder SH, ed. The encyclopedia of psychoactive drugs. New York: Chelsea House, 1985.

28. DSM-III-R Diagnostic and Statistical Manual of Mental Disorders (Third Edition-Revised), American Psychiatric Association, Washington, D.C. 1987, pp. 567.

29. Marrs-Simon PA, Weiler M, Santangelo MA, et al. Analysis of sexual disparity of violent behavior in PCP intoxication. Vet hum toxicol. 1988; 30: 53-55.

30. Howard J, Kropenske V, Tyler R. The long-term effects on neurodevelopment in infants exposed prenatally to PCP. In: Clouet DH, ed. Phencyclidine: an update. Washington, DC: Department of Health and Human Services, 1986, 237-251.

31. Luisada P, Phencyclidine. In: Lowinson JH, Ruiz P, eds. Substance abuse: clinical problems and perspectives. Baltimore, MD, Williams and Wilkins: 1981; 209-232.

32. Golden NL, Kuhnert BR, Sokol RJ, et al. Neonatal manifestations of maternal phencyclidine exposure. Perinat. med. 1987; 15:185-191.

33. Moerschbaecher JM, Thompson DM. Effects of phencyclidine, pentobarbital, and d-amphetamine on the acquisition and performance of conditional discriminations in monkeys. Pharmacol Biochem Behav 1980; 13:887-894.

34. Byrd LD, Standish LJ, Howell LL. Behavioral effects of phencyclidine and ketamine alone and in combination with other drugs. Eur J Pharmacol. 1987; 144:331-341.

35. Thompson DM, Moerschbaecher JM. Phencyclidine in combination with d-amphetamine: differential effects on acquisition & performance of response chains in monkeys. Pharmacol Biochem Behav. 20:619-627, 1984.

36. Wessinger WD, Balster RL. Interactions between phencyclidine and central nervous system depressants evaluated in mice and rats. Pharmacol Biochem Behav. 1987; 27:323-332.

37. Johanson CE, Balster RL. A summary of the results of a drug self-admin-

istration study using substitution procedures in rhesus monkeys. Bull Narc. 30: 43-54.

38. Yokel RA. Intravenous self-administration: response rates, the effects of pharmacological challenges, and drug preference. In: Bozarth MA, ed. Methods of assessing the reinforcing properties of abused drugs. New York: Springer-Verlag, 1987:1-33.

39. Overton DA. Applications and limitations of the drug discrimination method for the study of drug abuse. In: Bozarth MA, ed. Methods of assessing the reinforcing properties of abused drugs. New York: Springer-Verlag, 1987: 291-340.

40. Dorrance DL, Janiger O, Teplitz RL. Effect of peyote on human chromosomes: cytogenic study of the huichol Indians of Northern Mexico. JAMA, 1975; 234:299-302.

41. Ruffing DM, Domino EF. Effects of selected opioid agonists and antagonists on DMT- and LSD-25-induced disruption of food-rewarded bar pressing behavior in the rat. Psychopharmacology. 1981; 75:226-230.

42. Commissaris RL, Moore KE, Rech RH. Naloxone potentiates the disruptive effects of mescaline on operant responding in the rat. Pharmacol Biochem Behav. 1980; 13:601-603.

43. Carroll ME. Tolerance to the behavioral effects of orally self-administered phencyclidine. Dr Alc Dep. 1982; 9:213-224.

44. Nabeshima T, Yamaguchi K, Hiramatsu M, et al. Effects of prenatal and perinatal administration of phencyclidine on the behavioral development of rat offspring. Pharmacol Biochem Behav. 1987; 28:411-418.

45. Domino EF. Hallucinogens and inhalants. In: Drug abuse and drug research. The second triennial report to congress from the Secretary, Washington, DC: Department of Health and Human Services, 1987:183-213.

46. Spain JW, Klingman GI. Continuous intravenous infusion of phencyclidine in unrestrained rats results in the rapid induction of tolerance and physical dependence. J Pharmacol Exp Ther. 1985; 234:415-424.

47. Balster RL, Woolverton WL. Continuous-access phencyclidine self-administration by rhesus monkeys leading to physical dependence. Psychopharmacology. 1980; 70:5-10.

48. Schuster CR. Variables affecting the self-administration of drugs by rhesus monkeys. In: Vagtborg H, ed. Use of nonhuman primates in drug evaluation. Austin TX: University of Texas Press. 1968:283-299.

49. Balster, RL. Behavioral studies of tolerance and dependence. In: Seiden LS, Balster RL, eds. Behavioral pharmacology: The current status. New York: Alan R. Liss, Inc. 1985, 403-418.

50. Carroll ME. A quantitative assessment of phencyclidine dependence produced by oral self-administration in rhesus monkeys. J Pharmacol Exper Ther. 1987; 242:405-412.

51. Slifer BL, Balster RL, Woolverton WL. Behavioral dependence produced by continuous phencyclidine infusion in rhesus monkeys. J Pharmacol Exp Ther. 1984; 230:339-406.

52. Beardsley PM, Balster RL. Behavioral dependence upon phencyclidine and ketamine in the rat. J Pharmacol Exp. Ther. 1987; 242:203-211.

53. Wessinger WD. Behavioral dependence on phencyclidine in rats. Life Sci. 1987; 41:355-360.

54. Schlemmer RF Jr, David JM. A primate model for the study of hallucinogens. Pharmacol Biochem Behav. 1986; 24:381-392.

55. Kalant H, LeBlanc AE, Gibbins RJ. Tolerance to, and dependence on, some non-opiate psychotropic drugs. Pharmacol Rev. 1971; 23:135-191.

56. Lemaire GL, Meisch RA. Pentobarbital self-administration in rhesus monkeys: drug concentration and fixed-ratio size interactions. J Exp Anal Behav. 1984; 42:37-49.

57. Brady KT, Balster RL. Discriminative stimulus properties of phencyclidine and five analogues in the squirrel monkey. Pharmacol Biochem Behav. 1981; 14:213-218.

58. Carroll ME, Stotz DC, Kliner DJ et al. Self-administration of orally-delivered methohexital in rhesus monkeys with phencyclidine or pentobarbital histories: Effects of food deprivation and satiation. Pharmacol Biochem Behav. 1984; 20:145-151.

59. Beardsley PM, Balster RL, Harris LS. Behavioral dependence in rhesus monkeys following chronic THC administration. In: Harris LS. ed., Problems of drug dependence, 1984, Washington, DC.: US. Public Health Service, 1985, 111-117.

60. Carroll ME, Lac ST. Cocaine withdrawal produces behavioral disruptions in rats. Life Sci 1987; 40:2183-2190.

SELECTIVE GUIDE TO CURRENT REFERENCE SOURCES ON TOPICS DISCUSSED IN THIS ISSUE

Addiction Potential of Abused Drugs

James E. Raper, Jr., MSLS
Lynn Kasner Morgan, MLS

Each issue of *Advances in Alcohol & Substance Abuse* features a section offering suggestions on where to look for further information on topics discussed in the issue. In this issue, our intent is to guide readers to selected sources of current information on the addiction potential of abused drugs.

Some reference sources utilize designated terminology (controlled vocabularies) which must be used to find material on topics of interest. For these a sample of available search terms has been indicated to assist the reader in accessing suitable sources for his/her purposes. Other reference tools use keywords or free-text terms from the title of the document, the abstract, and the name of any responsible agency or conference. In searching using keywords, be

The authors are affiliated with the Gustave L. and Janet W. Levy Library, The Mount Sinai Medical Center, Inc., One Gustave L. Levy Place, New York, NY 10029-6574.

sure to look under all possible synonyms to get at the concept in question.

An asterisk (*) appearing before a published source indicates that all or part of that source is in machine-readable form and can be accessed through an online database search. Database searching is recommended for retrieving sources of information that coordinate multiple concepts or subject areas. Most health sciences libraries offer database services or searching can be done from one's office or home with subscriptions to database services and microcomputers equipped with modems.

Readers are encouraged to consult their librarians for further assistance before undertaking research on a topic.

Suggestions regarding the content and organization of this section are welcome and should be sent to the authors.

1. INDEXING AND ABSTRACTING SOURCES

Place of publication, publisher, start date, frequency of publication, and brief descriptions are noted.

Biological Abstracts (1926-) and *Biological Abstracts/RRM* (v.18, 1980-). Philadelphia, BioSciences Information Service, semimonthly. Reports on worldwide research in the life sciences.

> See: Concept headings for abstracts, such as behavioral biology, pharmacology, psychiatry-addiction.

> See: Keyword-in-context subject index.

Chemical Abstracts. Columbus, Ohio, American Chemical Society, 1907- , weekly. A key to the world's literature of chemistry and chemical engineering, including journal articles, patents, reviews, technical reports, monographs, conference proceedings, symposia, dissertations, and books.

> See: *Index Guide* for cross-referencing and indexing policies.

> See: *General Subject Index* terms, such as alcoholic beverages; drug dependence; drug-drug interactions; drug tolerance.

> See: Keyword subject indexes.

Dissertation Abstracts International. Section B. The Sciences and Engineering. Ann Arbor, Mich., University Microfilms, v.30, 1969/70- , monthly. Includes author-prepared abstracts of doctoral dissertations from 500 participating institutions throughout North America and the world. A separate section contains European dissertations.

See: Keyword-in-context subject index.

Excerpta Medica. Amsterdam, The Netherlands, Excerpta Medica Foundation, 1947- , 45 sections. A major abstracting service covering more than 4,500 biomedical journals. The abstracts, including English summaries for non-English-language articles, appear in one or more of the published subject sections, excluding Section 37, *Drug Literature Index*, and Section 38, *Adverse Reactions Titles*, which are indexes only. Each of the sections has a comprehensive subject index. Since 1978 all the *Excerpta Medica* sections have been available for computer searching in the integrated online file, EMBASE.

Particularly relevant to the topics in this issue are Section 40, *Drug Dependence*, and the sections that have addiction, alcoholism, or drug subdivisions: Section 30, *Pharmacology*; Section 32, *Psychiatry*; and Section 17, *Public Health, Social Medicine and Hygiene.*

Index Medicus (includes *Bibliography of Medical Reviews*). Bethesda, Md., National Library of Medicine, 1960- , monthly, with annual cumulations. Published as author and subject indexes to more than 2,500 journals in the biomedical sciences. Subject headings are based on the controlled vocabulary or thesaurus, Medical Subject Headings (MeSH). Since 1966 it has been produced from the MEDLARS database, which provides more comprehensive retrieval, including keyword access and English-language abstracts, than its printed counterparts: *Index Medicus, International Nursing Index* and *Index to Dental Literature.*

See: *MeSH* terms, such as alcohol, ethyl; amphetamines; anesthetics; barbiturates; benzodiazepines: cannabis; cocaine; hallucinogens; hypnotics and sedatives; marijuana abuse; morphine; narcotics, nicotine; opium; phencyclidine; rehabilitation; solvents; substance abuse; substance dependence; substance use disorders; tranquilizing agents.

Index to Scientific Reviews. Philadelphia, Institute for Scientific Information, 1974- , semiannual.

>See: Permuterm keyword subject index.

>See: Citation index.

*International Pharmaceutical Abstracts. Washington, D.C., American Society of Hospital Pharmacists, 1964- , semimonthly. A key to the world's literature of pharmacy.

>See: IPA subject terms, such as alcoholism, cocaine, dependence, drug abuse.

*Psychological Abstracts. Washington, D.C., American Psychological Association, 1927- , monthly. A compilation of nonevaluative summaries of the world's literature in psychology and related disciplines.

>See: Index terms, such as addiction, alcohol drinking attitudes, alcohol drinking patterns, alcohol rehabilitation, alcoholism, amphetamine, cocaine, drug abuse, drug addiction, drug dependency, drug interactions, drug usage.

*Public Affairs Information Service Bulletin. New York, Public Affairs Information Service, v.55, 1969- , semimonthly. An index to library material in the field of public affairs and public policy published throughout the world.

>See: PAIS subject headings, such as alcohol-and-youth, alcoholism, amphetamines, drug abuse, drug addicts, drugs, women-liquor-problem.

*Science Citation Index. Philadelphia, Institute for Scientific Information, 1961- , bimonthly.

>See: Permuterm keyword subject index.

>See: Citation index.

*Social Planning/Policy & Development Abstracts. San Diego, Calif., Sociological Abstracts, Inc., v.6, 1984- , semiannual.

See: Thesaurus and descriptors listed under *Sociological Abstracts*.

Social Work Research and Abstracts. New York, National Association of Social Workers, v.13, 1977- , quarterly.

See: Fields of service sections, such as alcoholism and drug addiction.

See: Subject index.

Sociological Abstracts. San Diego, Calif., Sociological Abstracts, Inc., 1952- , 5 times per year. A collection of nonevaluative abstracts which reflects the world's serial literature in sociology and related disciplines.

See: *Thesaurus of Sociological Indexing Terms*.

See: Descriptors such as alcohol use, alcoholism, drug abuse, drug addiction, drug use, health policy, substance abuse.

2. CURRENT AWARENESS PUBLICATIONS

Current Contents: Clinical Medicine. Philadelphia, Institute for Scientific Information, v.15, 1987- , weekly.

See: Keyword index.

Current Contents: Life Sciences. Philadelphia, Institute for Scientific Information, v.10, 1967- , weekly.

See: Keyword index.

Current Contents: Social & Behavioral Sciences. Philadelphia, Institute for Scientific Information, v.6, 1974- , weekly.

See: Keyword index.

3. BOOKS

Andrews, Theodora. *A Bibliography of Drug Abuse, Including Alcohol and Tobacco*. Littleton, Colo., Libraries Unlimited, 1977- .

Andrews, Theodora. *Guide to the Literature of Pharmacy and the Pharmaceutical Sciences*. Littleton, Colo., Libraries Unlimited, 1986.

Medical and Health Care Books and Serials in Print: An Index to Literature in the Health Sciences. New York, R. R. Bowker Co., annual.

See: Library of Congress subject headings, such as alcohol, cocaine, drug abuse, marihuana, narcotic habit, stimulants, tranquilizing drugs.

* *National Library of Medicine Current Catalog*. Bethesda, Md., National Library of Medicine, 1966- , quarterly, with annual cumulations.

See: *MeSH* terms as noted in Section 1 under *Index Medicus*.

Page, Penny B. *Alcohol Use and Alcoholism: A Guide to the Literature*. New York, Garland Publishing, 1986.

World Health Organization Catalogue: New Books. Geneva, World Health Organization, semiannual (supplements *World Health Organization Publications* and includes periodicals).

4. U.S. GOVERNMENT PUBLICATIONS

Monthly Catalog of United States Government Publications. Washington, D.C., U.S. Government Printing Office, 1895- , monthly.

See: Following agencies: Alcohol, Drug Abuse and Mental Health Administration; Food and Drug Administration; National Institute of Mental Health; National Institute on Drug Abuse.

See: Subject headings, derived chiefly from the Library of Congress, such as alcohol, cocaine, drug abuse, drug habit, drug utilization, drug dependence, drugs, marihuana, narcotics, opiods, pharmacology, stimulants, tobacco habit.

See: Title index.

5. ONLINE BIBLIOGRAPHIC DATABASES

Only those databases which have no print equivalents are included in this section. Print sources which have online database equivalents are noted throughout this guide by the asterisk (*) which appears before the title. If you do not have direct access to these databases, consult your librarian for assistance.

ALCOHOL AND ALCOHOL PROBLEMS SCIENCE DATABASE (National Institute on Alcohol Abuse and Alcoholism, Rockville, Md.).

Use: Keywords.

ALCOHOL INFORMATION FOR CLINICIANS AND EDUCATORS (Project Cork Institute, Dartmouth Medical School, Hanover, N.H.).

Use: Keywords.

ASI: AMERICAN STATISTICS INDEX (Congressional Information Services, Inc., Washington, D.C.).

Use: Keywords.

CRIMINAL JUSTICE PERIODICAL INDEX (University Microfilms International, Ann Arbor, Mich.)

Use: Keywords.

DRUGINFO AND ALCOHOL USE AND ABUSE (Hazelden Foundation, Center City, Minn., and Drug Information Service Center, College of Pharmacy, University of Minnesota, Minneapolis, Minn.).

Use: Keywords.

FAMILY RESOURCES DATABASE (National Council on Family Relations and Inventory of Marriage and Family Literature Project, Minneapolis, Minn.).

Use: Keywords.

LEXIS (Mead Data Central, Inc., Dayton, Ohio).

Use: Keywords.

MAGAZINE INDEX (Information Access Co., Belmont, Calif.).

Use: Keywords.

MEDICAL AND PSYCHOLOGICAL PREVIEWS: MPPS (BRS Bibliographic Retrieval Services, Inc., McLean, VA.).

Use: Keywords.

MENTAL HEALTH ABSTRACTS (IFI/Plenum Data Co., Alexandria, Va.).

Use: Keywords.

NATIONAL NEWSPAPER INDEX (Information Access Co., Belmont, Calif.).

Use: Keywords.

NTIS (National Technical Information Service, U.S. Dept. of Commerce, Springfield, Va.).

Use: Keywords.

PSYCALERT (American Psychological Association, Washington, D.C.).

Use: Keywords.

WESTLAW (West Publishing Co., St. Paul, Minn.)

Use: Keywords.

6. HANDBOOKS, DIRECTORIES, GRANT SOURCES, ETC.

Annual Register of Grant Support. Wilmette, Ill., National Register Pub. Co., annual.

See: Medicine; pharmacology; psychiatry, psychology, mental health sections.

See: Subject index.

Directory of Research Grants. Phoenix, Az., Oryx Press, annual.

See: Subject index terms, such as alcoholism, drug abuse.

Encyclopedia of Associations. Detroit, Gale Research Co., annual (occasional supplements between editions).

> See: Subject index.

Encyclopedia of Information Systems and Services. 8th ed. Detroit, Gale Research Co., © 1988.

Foundation Directory. New York, The Foundation Center, biennial (updated between editions by *Foundation Directory Supplement*).

> See: Index of foundations.

> See: Index of foundations by state and city.

> See: Index of donors, trustees, and administrators.

> See: Index of fields of interest.

Biomedical Guide to PHS-Supported Research. Bethesda, Md., National Institutes of Health, Division of Research Grants, annual.

> See: Subject index.

O'Brien, Robert and Sidney Cohen. *The Encyclopedia of Drug Abuse*. New York, Facts on File Pub., 1984.

Roper, Fred W. and Jo Anne Boorkman. *Introduction to Reference Sources in the Health Sciences*. 2nd ed. Chicago, Medical Library Association, © 1984.

The SALIS Directory: Substance Abuse Librarians and Information Specialists. Berkeley, Calif., Alcohol Research Group, Medical Research Institute of San Francisco and University of California, Berkeley, 1987-88, © 1987.

7. JOURNAL LISTINGS

Ulrich's International Periodicals Directory, Now Including Irregular Series & Annuals. New York, R. R. Bowker Co., annual (updated between editions by *Ulrich's Quarterly*).

See: Subject categories, such as drug abuse and alcoholism, medical sciences, pharmacy and pharmacology, psychology.

8. AUDIOVISUAL PROGRAMS

National Library of Medicine Audiovisuals Catalog. Bethesda, Md., National Library of Medicine, 1977- , quarterly, with annual cumulations.

See: *MeSH* terms as noted in Section 1 under *Index Medicus*.

Patient Education Sourcebook. [Saint Louis, Mo.], Health Sciences Communications Association, © 1985.

See: *MeSH* terms as noted in Section 1 under *Index Medicus*.

9. GUIDES TO UPCOMING MEETINGS

Scientific Meetings. San Diego. Calif., Scientific Meetings Publications, quarterly.

See: Subject indexes.

See: Association listing.

World Meetings: Medicine. New York, Macmillan Pub. Co., quarterly.

See: Keyword index.

See: Sponsor directory and index.

World Meetings: Outside United States and Canada. New York, Macmillan Pub. Co., quarterly.

See: Keyword index.

See: Sponsor directory and index.

10. PROCEEDINGS OF MEETINGS

Conference Papers Index. Louisville, Ky., Data Courier, v.6, 1978- , monthly.

Directory of Published Proceedings. Series SEMT. Science/Engineering/Medicine/Technology. White Plains, N.Y., InterDok Corp., v.3, 1967- , monthly, except July-August, with annual cumulations.

Index to Scientific and Technical Proceedings. Philadelphia, Institute for Scientific Information, 1978- , monthly with semiannual cumulations.

11. SPECIALIZED RESEARCH CENTERS

Medical Research Centres. 8th ed. Harlow, Essex, Longman, 1988.

International Research Centers Directory. 5th ed. Detroit, Gale Research Co., 1990-91, © 1990.

Research Centers Directory. 14th ed. Detroit, Gale Research Co., 1990 (updated by *New Research Centers*).

12. SPECIAL LIBRARY COLLECTIONS

Ash, L., comp. *Subject Collections*. 6th ed. New York, R. R. Bowker Co., 1985.

Directory of Special Libraries and Information Centers. 13th ed. Detroit, Gale Research Co., 1990 (updated by *New Special Libraries*).